Routledge Revivals

National Health Insurance in Great Britain

First published in 1946, *National Health Insurance in Great Britain: 1911-1946* by R.W. Harris provides a comprehensive analysis of the development and operation of Britain's National Health Insurance system. Divided into two parts, the book examines the scheme's foundations, administration, finances, and impact on society, as well as the evolution of the insurance medical service. It concludes with a forward-looking discussion on the transition toward a complete National Health Service. This work remains an essential resource for understanding the historical roots of Britain's health-care system.

National Health Insurance in Great Britain

1911-1946

R. W. Harris

Routledge
Taylor & Francis Group
ROUTLEDGE REVIVALS

First published in 1946
by George Allen & Unwin Ltd.

This edition first published in 2026 by Routledge
4 Park Square, Milton Park, Abingdon, Oxon, OX14 4RN

and by Routledge
605 Third Avenue, New York, NY 10158

Routledge is an imprint of the Taylor & Francis Group, an informa business

Publisher's Note
The publisher has gone to great lengths to ensure the quality of this reprint but points out that some imperfections in the original copies may be apparent.

Disclaimer
The publisher has made every effort to trace copyright holders and welcomes correspondence from those they have been unable to contact.

For Product Safety Concerns and Information please contact our EU representative GPSR@taylorandfrancis.com. Taylor & Francis Verlag GmbH, Kaufingerstraße 24, 80331 München, Germany

A Library of Congress record exists under LCCN: 46022108

ISBN: 978-1-041-28620-2 (hbk)
ISBN: 978-1-003-76559-2 (ebk)
ISBN: 978-1-041-28621-9 (pbk)

Book DOI 10.4324/9781003765592

NATIONAL HEALTH INSURANCE
IN GREAT BRITAIN
1911—1946

by

R. W. HARRIS

Chairman, Medical Service Sub-Committee
of the London Insurance Committee
Chairman of Appeal Tribunal
(Unemployment Assistance and
Supplementary Pensions)
and sometime Assistant Secretary
Ministry of Health

LONDON

GEORGE ALLEN AND UNWIN LTD

FIRST PUBLISHED IN 1946

Produced in complete conformity with the authorized economy standards

PRINTED IN GREAT BRITAIN
in 11 point Baskerville type
BY C. TINLING AND CO., LTD., LIVERPOOL, LONDON AND PRESCOT

FOREWORD (SEPTEMBER 1945)

This Enquiry was undertaken in the first instance, at the request of the Institute of Public Administration. It was substantially completed when the clouds of war were gathering and publication became impossible. The Institute thereupon left me free to make my own arrangements for publication when opportunity arose and for this I make my acknowledgments, and I should like to thank Sir Henry Bunbury and Sir Gwilym Gibbon for their patience before the war in reading the typescript; I am grateful, too, for the help given to me by a former colleague, Miss E. M. Foster, in the early stages of planning the book.

No extensive revision of the script has seemed to me to have been called for as the result of the working of the service under war-time conditions. but I have added a chapter to Part II to cover the progress of the negotiations, between the Government and the medical profession, on the establishment of a National Medical Service. The foreshadowing of such a service in chapter 14 and of a Ministry of Social Insurance in chapter 8, written two or three years before the appointment of the Beveridge Commission, has, it would seem, been justified by the march of events.

R.W.H.

INTRODUCTORY NOTE
(1938)

When in 1937 I undertook to prepare a research into National Health Insurance, the particular lines of research being left for me to decide, I must confess that I had not sufficiently realised what was in store for me. I have been engaged in National Health Insurance, in one way or another, since the day of the second reading of the Bill, in May, 1911; from one point of view, I know too much about the subject, and from another point of view, and that unfortunately covering many of the questions to which I should have to address myself in this paper, I have too little first-hand knowledge.

I gave much preliminary consideration to the question of the way in which the content of this paper should be circumscribed, e.g., whether I should attempt to cover the two fields of Health Insurance and Unemployment Insurance, with a view to establishing a comparison between the two, in regard particularly to the financial and administrative aspects. I surrounded myself with numerous books, reports and references, dipping first into one and then into the other, and in the result, I was able to delimit the lines of research in the manner indicated in the chapter headings. During the summer of 1937, there came into my hands, unexpectedly, five unpublished volumes of memoirs written by W. J. Braithwaite; and I am indebted to the reading of these memoirs for many of the memories, thus revived, of what happened in regard to the introduction of National Health Insurance.

I had only parted with these memoirs a few hours previously when the tragic news of Braithwaite's untimely death reached me. It was my sad privilege to contribute to *The Times* of 18th March, 1938, a short memoir about the man himself, and I have appended it to this introductory note.

I have thought that it would be of interest and of assistance in the consideration of the subject, if I wrote a short introductory note to each chapter, mentioning the sources of information on which I mainly relied in regard to the questions examined in that chapter, and adding notes of the books and publications in which the branch of the subject has been more extensively treated; so that those who may be especially interested in that branch of the subject, will know where to turn for a more complete exposition of the matter.

Apart from the human and social aspects of the National Health Insurance Scheme, Mr. Lloyd George clearly had in view in 1911 the economic aspect. He stressed on more than one occasion the importance to the employer of keeping the human part of his machine well oiled and well cared for, just as hitherto the mechanical parts had received attention.

Regarded as an organised scheme for securing payments during sickness and disablement to the worker the National Health Insurance scheme may be said to be generally accepted, everywhere, as an unqualified success.* I am not so sure about its contribution to the general health and welfare of the community. The medical provisions of the National Health Insurance Scheme have certainly secured to the worker a general practitioner service during sickness, and a new attitude of mind towards "calling in the doctor" and to the general practitioner a convenient and satisfactory method for securing payment for his services, but I think that the writer to the British Medical Journal, who recently said that National Health Insurance was a mere scratching of the surface, so far as the future of the medical service is concerned, was not far wrong. It is a matter of some concern that, after more than a quarter of a century of the working of this scheme, there have been no real developments in the direction of a complete and organised medical service.

I have, of course, devoted much attention to the report of the Royal Commission on National Health Insurance. So far as the cash benefits are concerned under the approved society system of administration, there was a general consensus of opinion in that report that the scheme had worked satisfactorily. The important recommendations in the Commission's report with regard to some developments of the medical services unfortunately came to no fruition. The report appeared at a time when nothing else in the

* The late Sir Alfred Watson, the Government Actuary, in his first report on the Valuation of Approved Societies, says "It will be seen how vast an instrument is National Health Insurance in affording protection to the industrial population against loss of wages during periods of incapacity for work." Later in the report he says "Taking the results as a whole no student of social conditions can fail to be impressed by the financial strength of the system of National Health Insurance and by the capacity of the system to minister to some of the most urgent needs of the industrial population."

country mattered except Economy with a capital E, and the few and comparatively inexpensive extensions of medical services which were recommended did not materialise.

It was in 1911 that I wes requested by the Chairman of the Board of Inland Revenue to go over to the Treasury and lend Braithwaite a hand with the National Health Insurance Bill which had just been presented to Parliament. I went, as a good official should. I found that most of the research and preparation which had been undertaken was the work of one man, W. J. Braithwaite, who had at hand a walking encyclopædia of information about the German system in the person of W. H. Dawson, to whose book on Social Insurance in Germany I shall make reference. I had none of Braithwaite's interest in Friendly Societies and, I fear, little of his enthusiasm. To me it was an unexpected piece of interesting work and very much of an adventure. We plunged along together in an atmosphere of deputations, interviews, conferences and correspondence, with an almost daily attendance at the House of Commons for a period of some months First one man came along from the Local Government Board, then one from the Admiralty, then two or three more from Somerset House, and so some sort of nucleus staff was built up against the day when the Bill should become an Act of Parliament and the new scheme would pass from the arena of Parliament into the field of administration. These months of 1911 represented a very exciting time, a tremendous scramble, with occasionally something of the feeling that one was taking part in a sort of Charge of the Light Brigade; ours not to reason why, but to get on with the job which Parliament in its wisdom was bringing into being. Now, after a quarter of a century, it is possible to look back and ask a series of questions, and in doing so, it seems almost inconceivable that some research into this amazing matter of National Insurance has not been essayed long before this.

It is my purpose to examine the foundations upon which this gigantic structure has been erected, what experience there was to guide Mr. Lloyd George and those who worked with him as to the possibility of the scheme functioning at all, and then as to the prospect of its functioning to the national advantage to an extent commensurate with the enormous burden of finance which was to be laid on different elements in the nation—the employer, the workman, and the State; followed by an examination of the administrative and financial problems presented by the Scheme considered as a *National Insurance* problem. This will constitute Part I of my paper. In Part II the medical provisions of the Scheme are considered as a contribution towards the very large and quite separate problem of *National Health.* I learned from Braithwaite's memoirs that, following the rather hurried passage of the Old Age Pension Act, 1908, and the appearance of the Poor Law Commission's report in 1909, Lloyd George was very active* at intervals on the subject of National Health Insurance. He received deputations from Friendly Societies and Trade Unions, and considered memoranda from the Registrar of Friendly Societies, the representatives of the various self-governing bodies, and from many other sources, and quite early, probably in 1909, he got as far as to say in public that he would prepare a scheme, and administer it through the Friendly Societies.

The time given to preparation and research was all too short; hustle was too predominant a factor. But if there had been the usual long period of preparation, with Royal Commissions and what not, before the scheme was embarked upon, it has seemed to many observers that we should never have had a National Health Insurance scheme at all. While that is to some extent right, that is not to say that the scheme was ill-advised and premature.

With reference to the element of haste there is an interesting parallel in the case of the social policy of Bismarck with regard to which a critical study was prepared by Miss Annie Ashley, of the University of Birmingham.† In the preface to that study Professor Gustav von Schmoller says: "An important factor in determining the scope and character of the whole body of insurance legislation was Bismarck's desire to carry out the great undertaking rapidly, and, in any case, during his own lifetime. When in the years 1882-5, a part of the scheme was presented for the consideration of the Prussian State Council, under the presidency of the Crown Prince, and Herr Botticher invited me to

* Lloyd George had been much impressed by the German scheme of Insurance and also he was curiously interested in the tuberculosis aspects of the matter. I say curiously, because the provision in the National Health Insurance scheme for dealing with tuberculosis, Sanatorium Benefit as it was called, was very soon to pass out of the insurance scheme, into the hands of the local authorities, where it should clearly have been placed at the outset—although it is fair to recognise that the attention given to the question of the treatment of tuberculosis under the National Health Insurance scheme served as an impetus which otherwise the local authorities would never have had.

† I have made extensive reference to this book in Chapter 2.

make a detailed examination of the Bill for extending accident insurance to the agricultural labourers, I expressed my doubt as to the advisability of such hasty legislation: in my judgment it would have been well to await the results of two or three years' experience of the recent combination of sickness and accident insurance in the case of the industrial workers. The answer I got was this: We cannot wait. Nothing but the force of Bismarck's personality will render success possible. If we lost him the work would be left half done."

I cannot do better than quote here a shrewd observation made by Sir Gwilym Gibbon in his paper on the Public Social Services read before the Royal Statistical Society in 1937. He says: "It is typical of the irony of history that Bismarck introduced sickness insurance, among other measures, partly to dish the social democrats, and in the result provided them with one of their best schools of administrative practice, and Mr. Lloyd George introduced a scheme of democratic administration which immediately became bureaucratic, though not governmental bureaucracy."

A few notes have been made on the moulding of the scheme embodied in the Bill, and on the starting-up of the machine, but this introductory note is already too long and I have embodied these additional notes in Appendix No. 1.

R.W.H.

MR. W. J. BRAITHWAITE

National Health Insurance

Mr. William John Braithwaite, C.B., died in the British Hospital, Port Said, on his way home from Burma, where, with his wife and daughter, he had visited his son. He was a brilliant Civil Servant, who had a large share in establishing the National Health Insurance scheme, and who also did a remarkable social work in Limehouse. A correspondent writes of him:—

> When in 1910 Mr. Lloyd George asked for a man to go along to the Treasury to help him with the National Health Insurance scheme, the chairman of the Board of Inland Revenue sent him a young assistant secretary, who had reached

that high position at the age of 36. He had much of the same quality of reckless enthusiasm as "L.G.", and more than a touch of genius. In a few months Braithwaite had, with practically no help at all, made a hurried study of the German scheme, visited various parts of the globe, and collected material enabling Mr. Lloyd George to produce his tremendous scheme, without a previous investigation by a Royal Commission, or a whole lot of Royal Commissions. In 1911, with just one or two to help him, he kept down the Chancellor's enormous post-bag, every day the correspondence, even from the humblest citizens, being answered somehow or other within 24 hours. He received hundreds of deputations, prepared notes on clauses, and spent hours of the day and night with Parliamentary draftsmen. In all the interviews with difficult organizations which had to be tackled, Braithwaite stood by the Chancellor and helped him to find a solution to every difficulty. Every member of the Government of that day and the heads of the Civil Service knew that the scheme was very largely Braithwaite's. The few months of rushed preparation and the intensive burden of the passage of the Bill through Parliament fell almost entirely on his shoulders, but recognition and honour at that time passed him by. The Companionship of the Bath, which was conferred on him last year, was a recognition of his years of service as a special commissioner of income-tax, to which office he was appointed at the end of 1912.

CONTENTS

Part 1. NATIONAL INSURANCE

Part 2. NATIONAL HEALTH

PART I

NATIONAL INSURANCE

PART ONE

NATIONAL INSURANCE

CHAPTER I

THE NATIONAL HEALTH INSURANCE SCHEME DESCRIBED

Note.

In the early days of 1912 it was decreed that there should be delivered by post at every house, cottage, and tenement in the land a paper which should tell every inhabitant of these Islands what his position was under the new scheme. It was the first such wholesale delivery that had ever been undertaken. It fell to my lot to draw up this leaflet. I put it through a series of ten proofs and tried twenty copies of each on all sorts of people, including maid servants. I passed the final proof for press on a Saturday morning and, on my arrival at the office on the Monday morning, I saw too late that the amount of the contribution was set out as sevenpence for men and sixpence for women, without any indication whether the payment was to be made daily, weekly, monthly, or just as the impulse moved the contributors. Most of the printing presses in London had run off between them twenty-five million copies during the week-end. Some retired admirals and generals wrote on their club note-paper, and asked that this slovenly document should be reprinted, and that the cost of reprinting should be deducted from the pay of the responsible official. I felt that this was a little hard, and I am glad that this was not done as I should have had no more pay for the rest of my life. It was common knowledge that the contributions were weekly contributions, and the matter had to rest there.

There lie before me leaflets No. 31 and No. 35, of 1944, issued by the Ministry of Health, in which the scheme of National Health and Pensions Insurance is expounded in popular language. These leaflets appear to me to be the lineal descendants of my original effort, and I have borrowed a description of the scheme from these leaflets.

(1) *Persons required to be insured*:

In general all persons of the age of sixteen or over, including married women, who are engaged in any employment under a contract* of service are required to be insured under the National Health Insurance and Widows', Orphans' and Old Age Contributory Pensions Acts if the employment is remunerated at a rate not exceeding in value £420 a year, or, where the employ-

* Certain persons not employed under a contract of service are also required to be insured, viz. persons employed under a contract for the performance of manual labour for the purposes of an employer's trade or business, outworkers, cab drivers, and fishermen and other seamen paid by the share.

ment is by way of manual labour, without any limit as to remuneration. Apprentices are required to be insured if they receive wages or other money payments in return for their services. Aliens are subject to compulsory insurance equally with British subjects.

Certain classes of employment are specially excepted from the compulsory provisions of the Acts, e.g. casual employment which is not for the purposes of the employer's trade or business, employment by parents without money payment and certain employments which are ordinarily adopted as subsidiary and not as the principal means of livelihood. Apart from these exceptions, the fact that an employment is temporary, or for part time only, does not affect the question of liability for insurance.

Juvenile Contributors. Boys and girls under the age of 16 who are employed in an insurable employment are required to have a health insurance contribution of 4d. paid in respect of them for each week during which they are employed. The contribution is payable by the employer, but 2d. is recoverable from the juvenile. In return for the contributions, juveniles are entitled to medical benefit but not to any other benefits and the contributions do not count towards satisfying the qualifying conditions for cash benefits after age 16.

(2) *Exemption.* (Provisions suspended during the war for new applicants.)

An employed person who so desires may obtain exemption from compulsory health insurance if he proves that he is (1) in receipt of a pension or private income of £26 a year or more, or (2) mainly dependent for his livelihood on another person, or on some occupation which is not insurable under the Acts. A person who obtains exemption is entitled under certain conditions to medical benefit, but to no other health insurance benefit. The employer is still required to pay his share of the ordinary contributions.

(3) *Contributions.*

Contributions to the National Health Insurance and Pensions Scheme are payable by combined health and pensions insurance stamps. The ordinary weekly rates of contributions* are men 2/-,

* The proportions of the ordinary weekly rates of contributions which are payable in respect of National Health Insurance are: men 11d. and women 10½d.

women 1/7d. Of the 2/- contribution for men, 1/- is normally payable by the employer and 1/- by the worker, by deduction from wages, and of the 1/7d. contribution for women 9d. is payable by the employer and 10d. by the worker. But the amount payable by the employer is more and the amount payable by the worker is less where an insured person aged eighteen or over receives remuneration which does not exceed 4/- for a full working day and does not include board and lodging. There are special rates of contribution for persons in the Mercantile Marine employed on foreign-going ships and for men serving in H.M. Forces.

(4) *Steps to be taken by insured persons.*

Every person who is required to be insured must obtain a contribution card for his employer to stamp, and his employer can demand its production at any time. It must be delivered to the employer on the commencement of employment and whenever he may reasonably require it for the purpose of paying contributions or for production to an inspector or other authorised person.

It is the employer's duty to stamp the card of the employee for the week in which the employee reaches the age of sixteen and for each week (Sunday midnight to Sunday midnight) during the whole or any part of which he is subsequently employed. The employer must in the first instance pay the full amount of the contribution and, provided he has stamped the card in the correct manner and at the prescribed time (i.e. before the time of payment of wages for the period for which the contributions are due) he may, in the case of persons between the ages of sixteen and sixty-five (sixty in the case of a woman) recover from the employee the appropriate proportion of the contribution. In the case of men aged sixty-five or over and women aged sixty or over special contributions are required to be paid by the employer, no part of the contributions being recoverable from the worker.

To obtain the full advantages of Health Insurance it is necessary for the worker to join an Approved Society. Rejection by an approved society does not relieve the person from liability to be insured. An insured person who does not join an approved society within a certain time becomes a "deposit contributor". For health insurance purposes the maximum amount he may receive by way of cash benefits is limited to a sum equivalent to

7d. for each contribution received in respect of him. A person who can shew in the early years of his insurance that he cannot gain admission to an Approved Society on account of his health may be admitted to a special Insurance Section of the Deposit Contributors Fund and thereupon becomes entitled to the ordinary benefits of the National Health Insurance scheme. The benefits of deposit contributors are administered through the Insurance Departments.

An insured person must surrender his contribution card at the end of its period of currency in accordance with the instructions printed on the card. At the end of its period of currency the insured person receives his card from his employer and is required to surrender the card, whether stamped or not, immediately to his society; otherwise serious loss of benefit may result. If a person is insured at any time before joining a society he should, in his own interests, give the society full information about his previous insurance, as he may be found to have already acquired some benefit rights.

Every insured person between the ages of sixteen and sixty-five (sixty in the case of a woman) is entitled to receive a membership record card from his society, or from the appropriate Insurance Department.

The payment of qualifying contributions.

Until 104 contributions have been paid since the entry or last re-entry into insurance an insured person may in certain circumstances stamp his card for weeks of genuine unemployment or of sickness, for the purpose of completing as soon as possible the qualifying number of contributions for sickness, disablement, or maternity benefit. Except in these circumstances it is not open to a person insured as an employed contributor to stamp his own card for weeks during which he is not employed.

Arrears of Contributions.

Sickness and Disablement benefits payable to members of Approved Societies during a benefit year (January to December) depend upon the number of contributions credited to the insured person for the contribution year terminating about the end of the previous June. If he is credited with a prescribed number of contributions during a contribution year he is entitled to full benefits during the benefit year commencing in the following January, and if the number of contributions credited for the contribution year falls below that number he is liable to a reduction or suspension of benefits unless he makes the appropriate arrears payment. The prescribed number of contributions for full benefit at the present time is fifty for each year. This prescribed number includes any contributions excused for periods of duly notified incapacity for work and a credit for each week of proved genuine unemployment.

Maternity benefit is not payable unless for the contribution year preceding the benefit year in which the confinement occurred, the contributor is credited with at least 26 contributions (paid or excused).

Health Insurance Benefits.

The ordinary benefits of National Health Insurance are:

(1) Medical Benefit, consisting of free medical attendance and treatment, medicines and certain medical and surgical appliances.

(2) Sickness Benefit, and

(3) Disablement Benefit; these being weekly payments at the rates set out in the table shown below during periods of incapacity for work.

(4) Maternity Benefit, being a payment of 40/- on the confinement of an insured woman or of the wife of an insured man.

Where its funds permit, that is to say, where there are available surpluses disclosed on valuation, a society may also provide additional benefits in the form of an increase in the rates for sickness, disablement, and maternity benefits, or payment of the whole or part of the cost of certain treatment, such as dental or ophthalmic treatment, or treatment in hospitals or convalescent homes. An insured person does not become entitled to additional benefits until a certain period has elapsed since he joined the society.

(A) *Sickness and Disablement Benefit.*

The ordinary rates of sickness and disablement benefit are as follows*: —

SICKNESS BENEFIT.	Men.	Unmarried Women and Widows.	Married Women.
(*a*) After 104 weeks in insurance and payment of 104 weekly contributions	18s. a week.	15s. a week.	13s. a week.
(*b*) After 26 weeks in insurance and payment of 26 weekly contributions but before the completion of the conditions at (*a*) above ..	12s. a week.	10s. 6d. a week.	10s. 6d. a week.
DISABLEMENT BENEFIT.			
After 104 weeks in insurance and the payment of 104 weekly contributions	10s. 6d. a week.	9s. a week.	8s. a week.

Sickness benefit commences on the fourth day of incapacity and may be paid for a total of 26 weeks. Periods of illness separated from each other by less than twelve months are added together for the purpose of calculating this period of 26 weeks, and benefit commences on the *first* day of any period of illness which is joined up in this way with an earlier period. Where there is an interval of twelve months or more since the last illness the 26 weeks of sickness benefit start afresh. On incapacity continuing after the 26 weeks of sickness benefit have been completed, disablement benefit becomes payable, if the qualifying conditions for that benefit have been satisfied, and remains payable during the continuance of the incapacity for work.

An insured person who is an inmate of a hospital, asylum, public assistance institution, or similar institution supported by subscriptions out of public funds, may not receive his sickness or disablement benefit until he is discharged from the institution, when it will normally be paid to him by instalments. If, however, he has any dependants, the benefit is payable to them or, if none, it may be paid, if he so desires, to meet expenses for which he is liable or to the institution.

Where an insured person has recovered or is entitled to recover compensation or damages in respect of an injury or disease, sickness or disablement benefit is not payable in respect of incapacity due to the injury or disease except in so far as the weekly value or weekly amount of the compensation or damages is less

* These benefits cease to be payable to men at age 65 and to women at age 60, when pension normally becomes payable.

Sickness and disablement benefits are subject to suspension or reduction where the incapacity is caused by war injury or disease for which a disability pension is awarded.

than the amount of benefit which would ordinarily have been payable. An Approved Society may in its discretion pay benefit by way of advance pending settlement of an insured member's claim to compensation or damages, such advances being recoverable out of the compensation or damages when received.

(B) *Medical Benefit.*

An insured person is entitled to this benefit immediately on becoming insured. He receives a medical card from the insurance committee for the area in which he resides and he is required to take this card to the insurance doctor of his choice as soon as possible. Any medicine necessary is normally obtainable on the doctor's prescription from a chemist, but in those areas, mainly the rural districts, where chemists are not easily available, it may be supplied by the doctor himself. If the insured person requires medical attention before receiving a medical card he should apply to an insurance doctor taking with him, if possible, a form Med. 50, obtainable from a Post Office. The doctor may charge a fee by way of deposit, for which he should give an official receipt, and if medicine is purchased on his prescription, a receipt should be obtained from the chemist. The receipts and prescription may be sent to the local Insurance Committee who have power to refund the amounts paid.

The service to which an insured person is entitled is treatment by a general practitioner; he is not entitled to specialist services or treatment in an hospital; nor does the service include treatment during confinement, for which a cash benefit is paid as maternity benefit. Every insured person is entitled to choose his own doctor from the list (or panel) of those doctors who have undertaken insurance medical service, and he is entitled at prescribed intervals to change his doctor. Similarly the doctor is entitled, under certain conditions, to refuse to accept an insured person, or to require to have a name removed from his list. The important duty devolves upon every insurance practitioner of furnishing certificates of incapacity to insured persons to enable them to claim the cash benefits from their societies.

(C) *Maternity Benefit.*

This is a payment on the confinement of an insured woman or of the wife of an insured man. A married woman who is insured is normally entitled to two maternity benefits, one from her own insurance and one from her husband's. If her husband is not insured, or benefit for any reason is not payable from his insurance, two benefits are payable from her own insurance.

Maternity benefit is not payable until after 42 weeks in insurance and the payment of 42 weekly contributions.

PENSIONS.

Although the subject of Pensions is outside the scope of the paper, a short note of the position is appended:—

The pensions provided by statutory authority are as follows:—

The Old Age Pension (first provided under the Act of 1908) granted at age 70 without any contribution. It is subject to means and residence tests.

The Contributory Pension, associated with the National Health Insurance scheme; i.e., pensions for insured men at 65 and insured women at 60, and for wives at 60 whose husbands are entitled to pension—with a title at age 70 to enter upon the old age pension, without any means test, test of residence, or nationality. The contributory scheme also provides for a pension for a widow until she reaches age 70—when it is replaced by a non-contributory pension irrespective of any test as to means, etc.; and provision for children up to certain ages.

Widows' Pensions and Old Age Pensions on a contributory basis to the "black coated worker"—under the Contributory Pensions (Voluntary Contributors) Act, 1937. The contributions in this case are not linked up with National Health Insurance.

Supplementary Pensions (including an allowance for dependants) granted by way of addition, where there is need, to an Old Age Pension or, in certain cases, a Widows' Pension.

APPENDIX 1 TO CHAPTER I.

A provisional scheme was formulated and referred to actuaries in 1910. The report of the actuaries is a confidential document of 49 blue book pages, a very careful and valuable paper, and it actually formed the basis for the finance of the bill, with the necessary modifications. No useful purpose would be served at this date by examining the provisional scheme in any detail.

Except that a scheme of pensions for widows and orphans was examined, the scheme differed very little in broad outlines from the one which was introduced into Parliament in 1911. The same general provisions are there, the compulsory scope of the scheme being broadly applied to all persons under contract of service, the limitation of persons not engaged in manual labour to those with an income of not more than £160 a year, provisions for the valuation of self-governing societies by a Government actuary and the audit of their accounts by Government auditors; special arrangements for any prospective losses to the fund being made good by the State, in one or other of three ways; protection of the funds of the old Friendly Societies and the right of self-management fully preserved, with a controlling central administrative body.

APPENDIX 2 TO CHAPTER I.

TEMPORARY PROVISIONS TO MEET WAR CONDITIONS.

Emergency legislation was passed in order, as far as possible, to adjust the schemes to war conditions. The main provisions of the relevant Acts are as follows:—

(i) *War Occupations.*

Special provisions are made to maintain the insurance rights of persons engaged in certain non-insurable occupations directly connected with the war, namely:—

(*a*) employment abroad which would have been insurable if the employment had been in Great Britain: under the Act this is treated as if it were insurable employment; and

(*b*) certain other non-insurable occupations in this country and abroad, *e.g.*, canteen work not under a contract of service, in respect of which, by paying contributions in respect of the war occupation, the worker may maintain the insurance in force when the occupation started.

The normal rates of pensions contributions are payable in respect of war occupation periods but, as the insured persons concerned are entitled only to limited health insurance benefits while engaged in the war occupation, the National Health Insurance contributions are reduced to 4d. for men and 3½d. for women.

(ii) *Auxiliary Forces of the Crown.*

Many persons (including women) are, during wartime, employed under the Crown under conditions similar to those of men of the Forces and provision is made for their health and pensions insurance on a similar basis.

The rates of contributions are:—

Health Insurance, Men 4d., Women 3½d. per week.

Pensions Insurance, the normal contributions.

(iii) *War Disability Allowances and Pensions.*

Special provisions are made with regard to the adjustment of benefits of persons who are entitled to pensions or allowances in respect of incapacity due to injury or disease attributable to or aggravated by the war. These persons are:—

(*a*) civilians (including masters and seamen in the Mercantile Marine) who sustain war injuries or war service injuries; and

(*b*) persons awarded pensions or grants on discharge from His Majesty's Forces or Auxiliary Forces.

In the case of civilians, etc., sickness benefits are not payable in respect of incapacity due to the injury or disease for a period of 26 weeks reckoned from the Monday preceding the date of injury, or, in the case of disease, from the date of first removal from duty.

In the case of persons discharged from His Majesty's Forces, the suspension from title to benefit for the first 26 weeks after the date of injury or removal from duty mentioned above, does not apply. Otherwise, the provisions are the same both for civilians and for persons discharged from the Forces.

After the expiration of the 26 weeks, if a pension in respect of disablement in the highest degree is awarded or if injury allowance continues, sickness benefit is reduced by half and disablement benefit is not payable.

Where pension is payable for partial incapacity, the rate of sickness or disablement benefit must be reduced, if necessary, to secure that the pension and benefit taken together do not exceed the total amount to which the person would be entitled by way of pension and benefit if he were in receipt of a highest degree pension.

The above restrictions cease to apply as regards reduction of sickness benefit after the insured person has been engaged during 26 weeks in insurable employment or some regular occupation and 26 contributions have been paid by or in respect of him since the date of the war injury, war service injury or the date of discharge as the case may be, and, similarly, as regards disablement benefit after 104 weeks in insurable employment or some regular occupation and the payment of 104 contributions.

CHAPTER II

FOUNDATIONS

(1) THE GERMAN SYSTEM.

Note.—For the information in this chapter, I have relied in the main upon the following works of reference :

The Social Policy of Bismarck. (Annie Ashley) Longmans, Green & Co., 1912.
Social Insurance in Germany. (W. H. Dawson) Fisher Unwin, 1912.
Memorandum on Sickness and Invalidity Insurance in Germany, C.D. 5678. 1911. H.M. Stationery Office.

A complete summary of the provisions of the Acts relating to Sickness, Maternity and Funeral benefits throughout the world will be found in Appendix D to the Report of the Departmental Committee of Enquiry into National Health Insurance issued by the Government of the Union of South Africa. (Pretoria, U.G. No. 41—1936).

A review of the most recent developments in the field of social insurance in the several countries is contained in an extract from the year book of the International Labour Office 1937-38 entitled *Social Insurance in* 1937, and issued at the price of 6d.

By the year 1911, when National Health Insurance was introduced into this country, most of the chief countries of Europe had already made some sort of provision for sickness, accident and old age in their legislation. Between the years 1883 and 1911, Austria, Belgium, France, Denmark, Italy, Norway and Sweden had passed various measures of social insurance, differing in form from the German scheme but all largely the result of German action. State socialism had caught hold of the minds of men. The Sickness Insurance Bill passed in Germany in 1883 under the Bismarck regime was amended from time to time in the years which followed, and it is of interest to note that the consolidating Bill in Germany, embodying all these various amendments, was passed in July 1911, just at the time when Parliament was struggling with the whole question in Great Britain for the first time. In examining the foundations on which the insurance scheme in this country was built, we have therefore to look closely into the history of German legislation and what preceded it.

When the question of workmen's insurance in Germany was receiving attention in 1881 and steps were taken to draft the measure which finally was passed in May 1883, the principle of mutual insurance was by no means a new one. In South Germany there was in the parishes a system of sick relief for servants and dependent labourers which was based upon the insurance principle. There were also, especially in the North, a great many benefit societies of different kinds. The most remarkable were those amongst the miners in the Hartz mountains. At first they were entirely in the hands of the workpeople who bore the entire cost. The men of each mine were as a rule separately organised, so that there was a group of independent societies. The rates of contribution and relief varied considerably. As time went on the system was more and more unified.

Two extremely important changes occurred. The first was the beginning of co-operation between master and men. Throughout their later history each society was managed by a committee, consisting half of masters and half of men, and both contributed, employers paying the whole sum and deducting each man's share from his wages. In the second place, in the time of Frederick the Great, membership became compulsory.

A mining law of 1867 made further reorganisations necessary. After great opposition from the Societies, which disliked all interference, statutes still further modifying and unifying the societies were passed in Prussia in 1869. The system was now uniform, though each society still managed its own fund. The benefits were: (*a*) A permanent pension in case of invalidity; (*b*) in case of death, a permanent pension for the widow, unless she married again; (*c*) help towards the education of the children of members who had died, or who were invalided, up to fourteen years of age; (*d*) doctor's care and medicine; (*e*) sick pay; (*f*) burial money.

These miners' societies were not the only societies managed upon the basis of mutual insurance. Among the others, the most notable were those formed by the guilds. About the year 1845, new trade laws appeared, and in these are to be found clauses recognising two types of sick association, the guilds and apprentice societies. The guilds were allowed to form sick, burial, and relief societies. The beginning of State compulsion (though as yet for the most part only theoretical) may be noticed in the provision that, except in the case of the higher grades of workmen, all who failed to join some society were required to account for this before the authorities. In 1854 a law was passed still further protecting the guild, but at the same time providing for the establishment of new societies in certain trades according to local regulations. These were compulsory, and employers were obliged to pay one half of the subscription.

It is of interest to note that, although the most fundamental difference between the national system of insurance against sickness and disablement adopted for the United Kingdom in 1911 and the corresponding statutory provisions then in existence in Germany, was that of organisation, the influence of the English Friendly Society movement is to be observed in the law which was passed in Prussia so long ago as 1854, empowering local authorities to require dependent workpeople to join benefit societies. Under this law a great increase in the provision for sickness took place. In 1874 it was estimated that 5,000 societies with a membership of 800,000, a revenue of £450,000 and accumulated funds of £650,000 existed in Prussia. By this time there had also come into existence a large class of voluntary aid or benefit societies. These were also formed more or less on the model of the English Friendly Societies. It was for the development of these that the Imperial Law of 1876 was passed, providing for registration, restricting the functions of such societies in the granting of sickness and funeral benefits, fixing the rates of contributions and benefits, and providing for the security of the funds.

The German Sickness Insurance Bill, as noted, was passed in May, 1883. The greater part of the discussion in the Reichstag ranged around the principle of compulsion. Amongst the other principles involved which, however, did not cause so much controversy, was that of universality. The adoption of the contributory principle was no mere accident; it was the method of the Imperial system, as it had previously been that of the voluntary societies. It was believed that by this method men could receive relief without lessening their self-respect and independence of spirit.

The German Insurance Consolidation Act 1911 extended and amended the sickness insurance legislation more than that relating either to accident or invalidity. The old catalogue of trades and occupations liable to insurance gave place to the following more comprehensive list:—

1. Workpeople, assistants, journeymen, apprentices, servants;
2. Works' officials, foremen, and other employees in a similar leading position, in so far as this employment formed their principal occupation;
3. Assistants and apprentices in shops and pharmacies;

4. Members of theatrical and orchestral companies;
5. Teachers and tutors;
6. Out-workers;
7. Crews of German sea-going vessels where not protected by the Merchant Shipping Act and the Commercial Code, and those engaged in inland navigation.

Certain classes of employees were exempted from liability to insurance, e.g. officials of the State, employed persons belonging to communal bodies and insurance authorities, teachers, etc., provided they had a claim on their employers equivalent to the sickness benefit provided by the law.

The new law aimed at greater centralization with a view to superseding small and inefficient funds. Two groups disappeared entirely—the parochial and building trade funds which accounted for more than one-third of all the funds in existence in 1910. The funds then recognised by law were as follows:—

1. General Local Funds;
2. Factory and Works Funds;
3. Guild Funds;
4. Miners' Funds;
5. Rural Funds;
6. Mutual Aid Funds.

The Miners' Funds were but little affected by the new law, which in this respect followed previous legislation. Formed for a special class of workpeople, subject to exceptional conditions and needs, and having behind them a long and unbroken record of invaluable service in the interest of thrift, they were left to do their own work more or less in their own way.

The benefits under the new law of 1911 were as follows:—

(*a*) Sickness benefit;

(*b*) Maternity benefit;

(*c*) Funeral benefit; and

(*d*) Family benefit.

(*a*) *Sickness benefit.*

This implied, as before, care in sickness from the beginning of the illness, comprising medical treatment and medicine, with spectacles, trusses, etc., for a maximum of twenty-six weeks. Sickness pay for the same period was the amount of half the basic wages for every work day during inability to work dating from the fourth day of sickness or the day of disablement if that was later. In the new law, the term 'inability to work' took the place of 'inability to earn a livelihood' with a view to defining more clearly what had been understood by the latter term. Inability to work was presumed when an insured person was either unable, or unable without risk of worsening his condition, to follow his usual occupation, independently of whether he might be able to do some other kind of work.

Although the law did not specifically require sickness funds to provide their members with dental service as a part of medical benefit, their power to do so was implied by a provision permitting them to conclude agreements with dentists if so disposed, and this power was widely exercised by the stronger funds. As an alternative to medical attendance at home, hospital treatment might be given.

(*b*) *Maternity benefit.*

This benefit (to the amount of the usual sickness pay) was payable for eight weeks, at least six of which must follow confinement, to women who had been insured for six months during the year preceding confinement; but the duration of this benefit could be reduced to four weeks in the case of female members of rural funds, who did not come under the Industrial Code, i.e. those engaged in agricultural or domestic service.

The duration of this benefit was originally three weeks following confinement; in 1892 the period was extended to four weeks, and in 1903 to six weeks. A further extension to eight weeks was provided for by the Insurance Consolidation Act of 1911. Confinement did not count as illness, however, and therefore did not of itself establish a claim to sickness benefits; if illness occurred, sickness pay and medical attendance might be claimed, but confinement and sickness pay were not granted concurrently.

(*c*) *Funeral money.*

The funeral money payable was twenty times the amount the

basic wages rate, and it was paid at the death of all insured persons, but also whenever death ensued within a year of the discontinuance of sickness benefit, so long as it was the result of the same illness and the deceased was to the last capable of working. By rule, however, the funeral money might be increased to forty times the basic rate.

(*d*) *Family benefit.*

This was an additional benefit given when a fund adopted a rule to that effect, and it might include medical attendance for members of an insured person's family not liable to insurance, maternity benefit to wives not liable to insurance, and funeral money on the death of the wife or husband or child of an insured person. Supplementary contributions would be levied on the insured persons where family benefits were given.

Special provisions applied in the case of a new class of insured persons brought within the scope of the law in 1911, e.g. domestic servants and agricultural labourers, casual labourers, itinerant workers and outworkers, seamen, etc.

Although, as stated, the British insurance scheme was based broadly upon the German scheme, the points of departure are very considerable and the complications to be found in the German insurance scheme have no counterpart in the British scheme. The British scheme deals with both sickness and disablement as part of a single transaction between the insurer and the insuring authority, and the twofold system of insurance is under one management. In Germany, on the other hand, sickness and disablement, the latter called invalidity, and provided for in conjunction with old age insurance, are dealt with by separate laws. An independent and wholly different system of administrative machinery is set up for each branch of insurance, and as the contributions are quite distinct, the contributors, both workpeople and employers, have to deal with two collecting authorities. The British insurance scheme provides for insurance, both against sickness and disablement, in approved societies, whereas in Germany workpeople are insured against these two contingencies in independent organisations. Sickness insurance, as already stated, is administered through funds or societies of six types. Invalidity insurance is administered by a number of pension offices formed on a territorial basis and by other institutions formed for special groups of employees, e.g. miners, state railway employees, and seamen.

With regard to the cost of sickness insurance in Germany, there was no Government grant in aid and the cost was borne, except in the case of the mutual aid funds, by the workpeople and the employers in the proportion of two-thirds and one-third respectively, though the employers usually bore a larger share in the case of the miners' funds. The contributions formed a certain percentage of the average wages. It was necessary as a basis of computation to divide the workers into wage-groups and a certain basis of assessment had to be devised so that the workers could be readily placed into the several groups; it is difficult to suppose that these typically German complications could ever be reflected in our own scheme, and no useful purpose would be served by setting out the range of contributions which fell to be levied under this complicated system, either so far as the workers or the employers were concerned.

The employers and workpeople bore the cost of invalidity and old age insurance in equal shares, the contributions being graduated according as the workman's wages fell into one of five groups.

It is necessary to mention the question of accident insurance, merely to say that in Germany the master is bound to insure against his workmen's accidents, whereas in England he is bound to pay compensation,* and usually finds it is wise to insure in a Company.

The total insurance charges on employers for sickness, accident,

* The Report of the Royal Commission on National Health Insurance (page 257) contains the following statement on the question of the inclusion of Workmen's Compensation in the National Health Insurance scheme :

"We examined Sir Walter Kinnear on this proposal, and we give the following extract from his reply :

'. . . The Department considers that it would not be practicable or desirable to merge the Workmen's Compensation Scheme in the Health Insurance Scheme . . . The risks covered by the Workmen's Compensation Act vary very greatly in various trades. These risks entail considerable variation in the rates of premium as between different occupations and a frequent revision of rates according to claim experience. I suggest that such a system could not be worked in conjunction with a general scheme of insurance based on flat contributions. If a flat rate of contribution were charged, it is suggested that such a system would be inequitable to the trades carrying the lighter risks, and would in any case remove from employers the incentive which at present exists to reduce the risk of accidents and thus secure a reduction in their premiums.'

We consider that the arguments advanced by Sir Walter Kinnear are conclusive on this subject, and we cannot recommend that the Health Insurance Scheme should be widened to cover the liability now provided under the Workmen's Compensation Acts."

and infirmity varied considerably betwen the several industries; the range appeared to be from 2·6 per cent. in the engineering industry, to as high as 8·2 per cent. in the coal mining industry.

The attitude of employers and workpeople towards the social insurance scheme in Germany, after long experience, must have had considerable influence in this country when it was decided to introduce a scheme of National Health Insurance. A review of the opinions of employers shows that, although there were necessarily a certain number who felt that the provision made for the worker by legislation tended to weaken in him the consciousness of his personal obligations to provide independently for himself and his family, the more general view was that the insurance law had exercised an enormously beneficent influence on the health, the standard of life, and the efficiency of the working classes. A prominent member of the tobacco trade and a member of the Reichstag, speaking in November 1907, said: "It is hardly possible to speak of these insurance contributions as constituting any special burden on industry, for if you regard the sum so paid, not as a percentage of wages, but of the year's turnover, it does not exceed one-half per cent. and in calculating the cost of goods that is the extent of the expense to be allowed for. That is so small a sum that it is neither right nor just to make a noise about it, and pretend that we can no longer pay it if our workpeople are to have increased benefits by new insurance legislation. Speaking honestly as one employer to another I am of the opinion that the investment in these insurance contributions is not a bad one."

Dr. Kauthmann, President of the Imperial Insurance Department, referring especially to accident and infirmity insurance, said, about the same time, "It must be acknowledged that the high expectations of the legislature have not been disappointed. The cost of insurance has been willingly borne by the employers, even those for whom it was not easy, while those who have given personal service in the work of administering the insurance scheme have gladly discharged their often laborious honorary duties. The sacrifice of the employers has gone much farther. In a spirit of magnanimity many of them have voluntarily extended the provision for their workpeople far beyond the requirements of the law."

It is a fair assumption that if the insurance laws had been found to be unremunerative and excessively burdensome German employers would not have been so ready as they were to supplement the benefits conferred by those laws by voluntary benevolence on similar lines; the welfare work done by many of the best known firms in the iron and steel, coal mining and engineering, chemical, textile and other trades, formed one of the most honourable chapters in the history of German industry.

With regard to the workpeople, Dawson says: "Obligatory insurance practised under State direction is only thrift systematised and protected by ampler guarantees than can be offered by private action and commercial enterprise. A fairly intimate knowledge of the German working classes in various parts of the country justifies the statement that these laws are regarded by them as constituting a social charter of labour." What made the German workmen specially attached to the laws was the knowledge that the benefits were a right and not a benefaction. This was not to say that the workpeople were contented. An employer writing at the time says: "It cannot be said that the insurance laws have created a more contented working class; even were the benefits under the insurance laws, great as they are, granted at the employer's expense, there would be no permanent satisfaction of the workpeople's wishes. The reason for this lies in human nature, and not in the law. When Bismarck proposed these laws, he said frankly that he did not expect to make the working classes contented, for in his view of human nature a perfectly contented man was a psychological impossibility."

It should be borne in mind that the references in this chapter to the German scheme are to the provisions of that scheme which obtained prior to the introduction of National Health Insurance in this country. The German scheme has, of course, from time to time undergone developments, but these are rather outside the purpose of this paper. Amongst the most recent may be noted the measure taken under the Act of 21st December 1937 with regard to the financial consolidation of the three schemes (workers', salaried employees' and miners') of invalidity, old age, and survivors' insurance. A further purpose of the Act was to set up a special family allowance fund for the insured population.

Under an order issued on the 6th September 1937 an important change was made in the Law relating to the formation of federations of insurance funds. These funds had by this date fallen into four groups—local, rural, works and guild funds. With a view to comparing their experience and adopting common measures for the protection of their entrants most of the funds in each of these groups had formed themselves spontaneously into a free federation, and the part played by these four federations in the successful operation of the insured scheme had increased steadily in importance. The Order of 1937, in making affiliation to the federations compulsory for all funds, conferred upon them the character of public bodies.

The work of simplifying the organisation in Germany of insurance has gone on from time to time, and it is noteworthy that there has been a substantial reduction of the number of separate sickness funds, which is comparable with the considerable reduction, to which reference is made elsewhere, in the number of societies administering the scheme in this country. Of the total number of sickness funds there were 4,565 at the end of 1937 as against 7,387 at the end of 1933.

Those who are interested in the various changes in social insurance in Germany and other countries would do well to refer to the International Labour Office publication, and as regards the most recent developments, should look at the pamphlet on *Social Insurance in* 1937, to which reference is made at the beginning of this chapter.

CHAPTER III

FOUNDATIONS

(ii) *The History of the Friendly Society—mainly of the Friendly Society movement.*

Introductory Note.

For this chapter I have relied mainly upon the following books :

The Law of Friendly Societies (edited by William Tidd Pratt and revised by Brabrook). Shaw and Sons, Fetter Lane, 1881.

Provident Societies and Industrial Welfare (Brabrook). Blackie and Son, 1898.

The Messenger Prize Essay on Friendly Societies (G. F. Hardy) C. & E. Layton, London, about 1888.

Friendly Society Finance considered in its actuarial aspects (A. W. Watson). C. & E. Layton, 1912.

A short guide on the historical and financial aspects of the *Manchester Unity of Oddfellows* published in connection with the 1934 Conference by the London A.M.P.A. Committee at their office in London.

The *Centenary Booklet* issued by the Ancient Order of Foresters, 1934, and the *Report of the Chief Registrar of Friendly Societies for the year* 1929, part 2, Friendly Societies, published by the Stationery Office as a blue book in 1931.

It is an arresting fact that a desire to provide members of the family with a good burial seems to have been the most potent form of provision which has been made throughout the ages, and that this very form of provision was excluded from the National Health Insurance scheme, for political among other reasons—to be replaced however at a later date by a more worthy and substantial form of provision, namely, that of widows' pensions and contributory pensions for the old age of the insured members.

In looking into the history of the provident movement one cannot fail to be struck with the prominence of this question of providing a burial benefit, death benefit, funeral benefit, or by whatever name it may be called. It has been observed already in the note with regard to the German scheme, and a short note of the position in our own country may not be out of place. The provision of burial money is an object that is very important to those whose income is too small to meet the expense caused by death in a family, and it is perhaps not surprising to find down the years this desire to render the last offices of respect to the dead, and to be saved the humiliation and indignity of having to leave to the parish the duty of burying the remains of those to whom they were attached in life. Prior to the coming into force of the National Health Insurance scheme the existence of this sentiment had resulted in the formation of societies* counting their members by the million, extending their operations over the whole of the United Kingdom, and employing an army of collectors. These societies were known as collecting societies, and all such as were registered after 1st January, 1896, were required to adopt "collecting society" as the last words of the registered name. The provisions of the Friendly Societies Act applied to such of the Societies as are registered under it, and those of the Collecting Societies and Industrial Insurance Companies Act, 1896, to all collecting societies, whether registered or unregistered, and to all Industrial Insurance Companies which receive contributions by means of collections on a similar system.

While this vast growth of the collecting societies is a matter of comparatively recent times, the provision of burial money is of great antiquity. We are here concerned with it in its bearing upon the Friendly Society movement. Amongst the traditions current in friendly societies' lodges, we believe there is to be traced an attempt to associate the modern Friendly Society movement with happenings as far back as the time of King Solomon. The rules of a Roman Burial Club in the time of Hadrian have come down to our own time. The members met once a month, and frequently dined together. They excluded from benefit any member who did not keep up his subscription, but when a member died who was not in arrears, they followed his body in a walking procession and paid the expenses of the funeral.

At least one Roman Club, the College of Smiths, is known to have existed during the Roman occupation of this country.

We have to come down to the thirteenth and fourteenth centuries in order to realise, in the setting up of the guilds of that time, some closer approximation to the more modern ideas of provision for those who were sick. A great social change was in progress. As regards the relief of the poor the first effect of the

* As an example of the beginnings of these collecting Societies, I give an extract from the Historical Sketch of the Royal Liver Friendly Society, which in 1937 had accumulated funds amounting to £25,000,000 :—

In the month of July of the year 1850, at a meeting of a few thoughtful working men, held at the inn known as "The Liver," St. Anne Street, Liverpool, it was decided to form a new burial club—burial clubs in those early days of primitive thrift being the chief methods in Liverpool of providing for the decent interment of the poor. They commenced with nine members, the name of the club being suggested by the sign of the house in which it was formed. It was registered on the 14th of August, 1850, as "The Liverpool Liver Burial Society," having its office at 14, Pickop Street, Liverpool.

change was that part of the functions hitherto performed by the Church were taken over by smaller communities of persons, each community or guild, as they were called, having a more or less distinct and well-defined object. These guilds undertook, though usually as an object of secondary importance, the distribution of relief among their members—this constituting them the first Friendly Societies in this country of which we have any clear information. They appear to have flourished up to the time of the Reformation, and most of them had provisions for the optional relief, by way of charity, of those members of the guild who were in want.

The following paragraph in the statutes of the Guild of Smiths, of Chesterfield, is of great interest.

> "When a brother is ill and needs relief, then he shall receive half a dime daily; when brethren fall into poverty then they shall go singly on certain days to the houses of their brethren, where each one shall be received civilly and he shall obtain whatsoever he may need in the shape of food and clothing as if he were the master of the house himself, and he shall also receive half a dime like those who are ill, and then he shall go his way in peace."

It is to these guilds that we look, rather than to the protective trade guilds which then existed, for the progenitors of our modern friendly societies. As to their financial basis we find that in some cases the contributions were equal, while in others they varied according to the means of the member, each contributing as much as he could to the common fund, not distinctly for his own benefit but for the benefit of the members generally or the community at large.

The following list of the provident objects of the mediæval guilds has been compiled:—

1. Relief of poverty.
2. Relief of sickness.
3. Relief in old age.
4. Relief on loss of sight.
5. Relief on loss of limb.
6. Relief on loss of cattle.
7. Relief on fall of a house.
8. Relief on making pilgrimages.
9. Relief in case of loss by fire.

10. Relief in case of loss by floods.
11. Relief in case of loss by robbery.
12. Relief in case of loss by shipwreck.
13. Relief in case of imprisonment.
14. Relief for defence at law.
15. Relief of the deaf and dumb.
16. Relief of the afflicted with leprosy.
17. Dowries on marriage of females, or their entering a house of religion.
18. Aid in temporary pecuniary difficulties.
19. Aid to obtain work.
20. Repair of roads and bridges.

The list is even more comprehensive than that in the Friendly Societies Act, 1896; it seems to include every possible ill that man is heir to, especially when it is remembered that these provident funds were largely supplemented by works of charity.

Brabrook, however, gives it as his view that the evidence of any direct connexion between the guilds of the Middle Ages and the modern friendly society is scanty, if indeed there can be said to be any such evidence at all.

Amongst the oldest societies now existing, are those founded in 1687, 1703, and 1708, among the Huguenot workmen in Spitalfields, and the modern London friendly society is one of the boons conferred by them upon the country in return for the hospitality extended to them. The Huguenots, expelled from France, found a home in England, only to find that as aliens they were debarred from the benefits of Queen Elizabeth's Poor Law. To meet the difficulty, they founded benefit societies, a few of which in the neighbourhood of Bethnal Green were in existence until quite recently. A complete list of the benefit societies which have been in existence for 100 years or more, and were still in existence, is given in the Report of the Chief Registrar of Friendly Societies for the year 1929. Nine of the Societies can claim to be more than two hundred years old, and twenty others more than 150 years old. The earliest societies still in existence, which are included in this record are: The Incorporation of Carters, in Leith, established in 1555, with 68 members at the end of 1928; The United General Sea Box of Borrowstounness, established in 1634, with 36 members in 1928, and the Fraternity of Dyers in Linlithgow, established in 1670, with 30 members at the end of

1928. Most of the old friendly societies in this list are accumulating societies which insure sickness benefit and sums at death of members and their wives. A few are dividing societies, but not of the common annual dividing type, and, with two possible exceptions, only commenced to divide part of their funds when they had accumulated large reserves.

Friendly society legislation in this country dates from 1793, and the first Friendly Societies Act was introduced partly with a view to relieving the public of some of the burden of poor relief. Friendly societies, had, at the date of the first Friendly Societies Act, been in existence in Great Britain for more than a century, and for even longer in Scotland, where the earlier societies, of which some are still in existence, were possibly isolated survivals of trade guilds. The operations of friendly societies had been much hampered by the lack of any legal status or protection of their members' interests, and the Act of 1793 led to the formation of a large number of new societies. The friendly societies existing at the close of the eighteenth century appear to have been very similar in the nature of their operations to those of to-day. It is difficult to estimate with any degree of certainty the number of societies or their aggregate membership. There is good reason for believing that they were at least as numerous in proportion to the population as at the present time. It was estimated in 1796 that the number of societies in London was 600, with a membership of 70,000, and five years later an estimate was made that in the whole kingdom there were 7,200 societies, with a membership of over 600,000.

The propriety of limiting the age at entry was very generally recognised, especially amongst those societies confining their membership to distinct trades or classes, and endeavours were often made to secure the permanency of societies by making the amount of the benefits depend upon the funds in hand. The provision for death benefit by means of levies upon the members at each death, no doubt a method of great antiquity, was also common, while there were provided in many societies pensions for the widows of members rather than funeral allowances.

The 1793 Act "For the encouragement and relief of Friendly Societies" defined Friendly Societies as societies for raising by voluntary subscriptions of the members separate funds for their mutual relief and maintenance in sickness, old age, and infirmity. The preamble affirms that the protection and encouragement of such societies would be likely to be attended with very beneficial effects, by promoting the happiness of individuals and at the same time diminishing the public burden. The public burden which the framers of the statute had in mind was no doubt that of poor law relief. The reform of the Poor Law in 1834 undoubtedly led to the formation of friendly societies, but it is another thing to say that the societies saved so much in poor rate. That would be to imply that their members, if they had not belonged to such societies, would have been destitute. Brabrook says that this would have been a libel upon the friendly societies' members; if they had not invested their savings in friendly societies, they would presumably have invested them elsewhere. A former secretary to the Ancient Order of Foresters, in his testimony before the Royal Commission on the Aged Poor, said that out of the half million of members who constituted that society, he could not find that there were as many as a hundred persons in receipt of relief under the poor law. This is the more remarkable in that the society itself did not insure, in the generality of cases, relief in old age, as such; it only granted sick allowance to an aged member when suffering from some disease which disabled him from work, and even then the allowance after short terms of full and half pay was reduced to quarter pay. If a society does not directly insure a member against pauperism in old age, the explanation of the reason for his not becoming a pauper is to be found in the moral character of the man himself. The considerations which induced him to belong to a friendly society are the same considerations which keep him independent of public aid in his old age.

On the 12th July, 1819, an act was passed, "for the further Protection and Encouragement of Friendly Societies, and for preventing Frauds and Abuses therein." It recited that the "habitual reliance of poor persons upon parochial relief, rather than upon their own industry, tends to the moral deterioration of the people and to the accumulation of heavy burthens upon parishes; and it is desirable, with a view as well to the reduction of the assessment made for the relief of the poor as to the improvement of the habits of the people, that encouragement should be afforded to persons desirous of making provision for themselves or their families out of the fruits of their own industry. By the contribution of the savings of many persons to one common fund the most effectual provision may be made for the casualties affecting all the contributors; and it is therefore desirable to afford further facilities and additional security to persons who may be willing to unite in appropriating small sums from time to time to a common fund for the purposes aforesaid, and it is desirable to protect such persons against the effects of fraud or miscalculation."*

The preamble went on to recite that the provisions of preceding Acts had been found insufficient for these purposes, and great abuses had prevailed in many societies established under their authority.

The main object of legislation for some years, following the Act of 1819, was to encourage the formation of sound societies, but many difficulties were encountered in achieving this object. The Act of 1819 required that the tables of Friendly Societies should be approved by "two actuaries or other persons skilled in calculation." This provision, however, was of little avail because the certifying justices accepted village schoolmasters as persons skilled in calculation. After ten years' trial the provision was abandoned and the justices themselves were left to decide as to the safety of the tables which a society proposed to adopt, although a public official (in England the barrister-at-law appointed to certify the rules of Savings Banks) was appointed to certify that the rules of friendly societies were in conformity with the law before they were confirmed by the justices. The Act of 1834 relieved the justices from any responsibility for the safety of tables, but the barrister was required to see that the rules were "calculated to carry into effect the intention of the parties framing them."

The Act of 1846 provided that the tables of a society must be approved by an actuary before its rules could be certified. This provision aroused dissatisfaction owing to the divergent views of actuaries in devising satisfactory tables for the use of societies. This divergence, as was subsequently demonstrated, was not the fault of the actuaries, but was due to the lack of accurate information as to the sickness and mortality rates prevailing in friendly societies. Provision had been made for the collection of such information by the Act of 1829, but no tables based on the information were published until 1845. In 1850, it was decided to allow societies, if they chose, to enjoy the benefits of the act as "registered" instead of "certified" societies, without approval

* It will be observed that, although the problem of how to keep a society sound was realised by the legislature from a very early time, the expedient of a periodical valuation was not adopted till the Act of 1875 was passed.

of their tables. In 1855 the distinction between "certified" and "registered" societies was abandoned as unworkable. An exhaustive inquiry was made into friendly societies by a Royal Commission appointed in 1871, and as a result of its report the Act of 1875 allowed friendly societies to be registered without any stipulation as to the safety of their tables (except in the case of societies providing annuities) and required instead that their financial position should be reviewed once in five years by a valuer, unless the Registrar decided that a valuation was not applicable to their operations. The general position has not been altered by subsequent legislation.

By the Act of 1875, by which friendly societies are now governed, the laws were both consolidated and amended. The following provisions of the new Act are among the most important:

The maintenance of the voluntary principle, as respects registration and the actuarial certification of tables.

The continuance of the quinquennial and annual returns.

The limitation of benefits, especially for infants' assurances, this provision also applying to industrial assurance companies.

The Treasury to issue regulations from time to time, and a power conferred on the registrars to appoint inspectors, when duly requested, to enquire into the management of societies, and to call general meetings of members.

The compulsory valuation of all registered societies every five years, and provision for the appointment of public valuers by the Treasury.

The reconstruction of the Registry Office, resulting in the appointment of an actuary to the Registry.

It seems desirable to supplement this general account of the history of the friendly society movement and of the legislation which governs it by a short account of the history of the Manchester Unity of Oddfellows. This history is of peculiar interest, and may be regarded as appropriate to this volume by reason of the fact that the Oddfellows produced in the actuarial world a star of the first magnitude—Alfred William Watson, upon whose review of the sickness experience of the Manchester Unity the whole financial structure of the National Health Insurance Act was based.

In 1808, Robert Naylor, who was Grand Master of the Oddfellows in 1832, started a social and benevolent club at the Ropemakers' Arms, Chapel Street, Salford. It was very successful and it was soon joined by a large contingent of members from the Prince Regent Lodge of Oddfellows of the Sheffield United Order. The Board of Directors of the Oddfellows decided that the date of the first meeting of this amalgamated society, which was held in the Robin Hood Hotel, Manchester on October 10th, 1810, is the first day of the Order. The Unity of Oddfellows, therefore, had its origin in a free and easy Salford Tavern. Its principal attraction was an initiation ceremony, or as it was more generally known, a "making." This Lodge of Naylor's, now known as the Abercrombie, and a few others, including Oddfellows' lodges in some tavern societies which had thrown in their lot with the Abercrombie, thought that the lodges could be something more than mere convivial associations. They were probably, too, suffering from the competition of the public house burying societies which were springing up all around, and so in 1813 they held a convention at which they decided to become a burying society with a funeral fund and to call themselves the Independent Order of Oddfellows under the Manchester Compliance. The word Unity made its appearance later. Thus the introduction of the funeral benefit marked the beginning of the existence of the Order as a friendly society.

At the close of the eighteenth century, as already noted, it was estimated that there were some 7,200 societies with a membership of 600,000. In the provinces every village ale-house sheltered one or more beneath its roof. In the British Museum the rules of upwards of 100 of these societies dating from 1750 to 1820, all centred round Newcastle-on-Tyne, are to be found. At Nottingham, in 1794, fifty-six friendly societies took part in the annual procession. The Act of 1793 speaks of friendly societies as being societies of good fellowship, and it was to meet the competition of these societies that the Manchester Unity began first of all with a funeral gift, then a sick gift, and finally gave definite funeral and sick benefits. If earlier history is to be examined for the origin of the Manchester Unity of Friendly Societies, it will be found that the mother lodge, in common with some other societies, possibly owed its origin to a resolution of the Grand Lodge of Freemasons, passed in 1724, which prohibited Freemasons from belonging to more than one London lodge. The first Oddfellows lodge made its appearance about 1736, and an Oddfellowship lodge established in 1748 was a London tavern society restricted to professional and well-to-do classes. Working men were excluded. It was a convivial society which from time to time made benevolent grants. It was not a friendly society. The legislation introduced in the closing years of the eighteenth century to stamp out revolutionary societies effectively broke up the Oddfellows, the prosperous members joining the Freemasons. A few lodges were carried on by working men who had gradually crept into the society. The industrial revolution led to a migration northwards, and in Lancashire and Yorkshire the Oddfellows entered on a new lease of life, and, as we have seen, the 10th October, 1810, is regarded as the birthday of the Manchester Unity. To-day the Manchester Unity of Oddfellows makes claim to be the largest, richest, and most helpful friendly society in the world.

The largest bodies amongst the friendly societies being the affiliated orders, and the two greatest of these the Manchester Unity of Oddfellows and the Ancient Order of Foresters, it seems fitting that a short historical account of the Foresters should also be given.

The Ancient Order of Foresters as it is known to-day commenced its activities during the reign of William IV in the year 1834. Its "dispensations" or official authorities through open court are stated to have been founded from time immemorial. Whatever justification there may or may not be for this claim to extreme antiquity it is certain that the present Order is the outcome of an earlier one known as the Royal Order of Foresters, a court of which was in existence in Leeds in the year 1790. Other courts of that Order were scattered over Yorkshire, Lancashire and Cheshire, and there was one in America. Originally these courts were little more than social clubs, but the process of time converted them into "burying societies" providing also "sick gifts" in cases of distress. Court No. 1 of the Royal Order changed its name from Perseverance to Court of Antiquity, and attempted, in virtue of a right which it claimed, to exercise authority over the remainder of the courts of that Order. Owing to the opposition which this attempt created, disruptive elements began to make their appearance. A meeting of courts which were opposed to putting into practice the new code of rules drawn up by this Court of Antiquity was held, and a resolution was passed to secede from the Royal Order. There came into being the Ancient Order of Foresters Friendly Society, which by the end of October, 1834, had 294 courts. The first High Court at this Ancient Order was held in the Salford Town Hall in August, 1835. It was attended by 285 delegates and the number of members at that time was estimated at 16,500. A revised initiatory ceremony was approved by the Manchester High Court at this time. The ceremony contained many elements of religious significance. Candidates for membership were required to undergo tests of courage by defending themselves with swords against any member in the court room; cudgels were substituted for swords at a later date. When the combat ended the Chief Ranger enlightened the candidate as to its meaning, stating that it was symbolical of the fight which all good Foresters should wage against the world, the flesh, and the devil.

The early members of the Order commenced all their proceedings with prayer. There were four authorised lectures entitled respectively, the Introduction; the Initiation; the Installation; and the Illustration, all of which contained many biblical allusions. Very few early Foresters could read. Lecture classes were formed at which a lettered member would read the lectures, and those unable to read would commit them to memory. In those days of first fervour the recital of the lectures was very popular, and it was no uncommon sight to see numbers of Foresters seated around another Forester listening to the lectures and to his explanation of the ceremonies. With the spread of general education the necessity for such meetings passed away.

The first ten years of the Ancient Order of Foresters was a period of extreme difficulty for the early leaders of the Order. The organisation grew rapidly and in haphazard manner, but its promoters were inspired by lofty ideals and were imbued with much zeal for those ideals. The members who thought and wrote and spoke at that time had ideas to which they could scarcely give coherent expression. They had a burning desire to improve the Order and yet they seemed to be struggling in the dark. Since 1843 the tone of thought has been more practical, the rude lessons which experience in the management of the Order gave the leaders having cooled their somewhat romantic ardour. At the time of the passing of the Friendly Societies Act, 1850, neither the Order nor its branches had any legal status; indeed they were definitely classed as illegal organisations. Their inclusion in this humiliating category was due solely to the fact that there were in use passwords and secret signs. They were thus brought within the ambit of an eighteenth century act directed against secret societies which had been passed subsequent to the date of the first Friendly Societies Act.

As the result of the report of the Royal Commission on Friendly Societies, and the passing of the Friendly Societies Act 1875, the constitution of affiliated orders, such as the Ancient Order of Foresters, received complete recognition. The Order's development during the last half-century has been mainly in the direction of financial consolidation.

It has been thought desirable to give a fairly full account of the early history of the Oddfellows and the Foresters, with their picturesque ceremonies and their ideals of self-help and self-government because it was originally conceived that these ideals were to be preserved in the administration of the National Health Insurance Scheme, an idea which had to be very early abandoned. But the disappearance of the old spirit which actuated these lodges and courts and also the fading-out of a great range of small societies not connected with an affiliated order, must not be attributed wholly or even mainly to the National Health Insurance Act; the trouble had set in long before.

It is true that the introduction of State Insurance immediately led to an accession to the ranks of the accumulative friendly societies of a large number of members who regarded their membership solely in the light of an insurance contract. They had no interest in their society as a club and the majority of them never attended their lodge meetings after the date of their initiation. That the decline of interest in lodge affairs, however, is not entirely new is suggested by the fact that as far back as June, 1848, a letter was addressed to the Editor of the *Odd Fellows' Chronicle* drawing attention to the bad attendance at lodge meetings. In those days, apparently, the reasons adduced included "the Hosts' keeping indifferent liquors," "smoking, and long discussions upon matters of business" and "the decline in the practice of giving testimonials to Past Officers." In these days the poor attendance at lodge meetings, even among the old members, may be attributed in large measure to the multiplication of counter-attractions and to other more intangible causes.

It has always been an article of faith amongst members of the accumulative friendly societies that—to use a phrase culled from the initiation charge used in one of the affiliated orders—membership involved "more than a mere monetary contract." The societies existed also—and in many cases even primarily—for social intercourse; they were in fact *friendly* societies. As such they were compact social organisations which wielded a powerful though unobtrusive influence. Quite apart from the direct functions of visiting and relieving their sick members, attending the obsequies of their deceased brethren and granting assistance to their widows and orphans, they were social clubs in which many men received an important part of their education, developed a capacity for civic service, learned the lessons of mutual help and thrift and in the process developed a sturdy independence. They guarded jealously their rights to govern themselves and resisted strenuously all encroachments upon their local autonomy.

The increasing emphasis upon the monetary contract aspect of friendly society membership and the growing aversion of the ordinary member from active participation in the affairs of his lodge have, not unnaturally, been accompanied by a tendency among accumulative societies to attach more and more importance to types of benefits in which the individual member secures far greater control over his personal contributions. It is the demand for this type of benefit which accounts for the remarkable growth of deposit and dividing societies to which we shall have occasion to refer. This in turn has led accumulative societies, in order to attract new members, to adopt tables of benefit somewhat similar to those issued by these other societies. Curiously enough, concurrently with this tendency of accumulative societies to borrow from the methods of deposit and dividing societies, those societies have returned the compliment by exhibiting a growing concern as to their actuarial soundness and have shown an increasing desire to buttress their financial position by the building up of reserve funds. It will be convenient at this point to indicate briefly the distinguishing features of the various types of society concerned.

CHAPTER IV

(*a*) TYPES OF SOCIETIES

(*b*) EFFECTS ON MEMBERSHIP AND FUNDS

Introductory Note.

In addition to the publications referred to in the introductory note to Chapter 3, I have made use of the following additional documents :—

(*a*) A paper on Friendly Societies since the advent of National Health Insurance, by Victor A. Burrows, F.I.A., F.S.S., published in the Journal of the Institute of Actuaries, Vol. LXIII, Part III, No. 307, for 1932.

(*b*) Several reports of the Chief Registrar of Friendly Societies (in addition to that for the year 1929).

(*c*) The five reports of the Government Actuary on the Valuations of Approved Societies, and

(*d*) A good deal of information given me at first hand by secretaries of the largest Societies.

In addition, the tabular statement giving the figures of membership of the various Societies for 1910 and 1934, and also particulars of the benefits paid and of the total funds of the Societies as at these dates respectively has been prepared from material supplied to me by the Chief Registrar of Friendly Societies, and I wish to make my sincere acknowledgments for the help that I have received at the Registry in this, and in many other ways.

(*a*) *Types of Societies.*

Before examining the different types of friendly society, as that term is generally understood, it is perhaps necessary to say a word or two about the history of trade unions, which also came into the administration of the National Health Insurance Scheme.

Brabrook examines the question whether a trade union is a provident society. He comes to the conclusion that if a society enables you to devote a portion of your wages towards providing for the future it is a provident institution. A combination which has the object of seeing that you get sufficient wages to pay your contributions to that society must also be provident. Apart from this, trade unions have to a large extent made definite provision against sickness, accident, and old age.

Trade unions are institutions of great antiquity; the trade guilds of the middle ages were trade unions. These guilds are now represented in London by the wealthy City companies, and their objects and operations have changed with the times, but many of them still bear in their charters and bye-laws traces of the trade regulations which formed a great part of their original object.

The primary and paramount object of a trade union is its trade object; if it be a workmen's union, the provision of funds that can be used, if the need arises, to resist on the one hand any attempt of the employers to lower the scale of wages or to render the conditions of labour more severe, or to help forward, on the other hand, any efforts on the part of the workmen to raise the scale of wages or to render the conditions of labour more lenient; if it be an employers' union, the converse. Workmen's unions, especially those of the older type, combine with this object other purposes, akin to those of a friendly society, such as relief in sickness, assistance towards emigration, and provision for funeral expenses at death. In ordinary times when no trade conflict exists the expenditure on these purposes largely exceeds the expenditure on trade purposes; for example in the year 1890, when the total expenditure of 259 trade unions, registered and unregistered, was £862,000, only £107,000 was spent in dispute benefits. Of the remainder, £173,000 was spent in sick pay and medical attendance, £145,000 for out-of-work benefits, £87,000 for superannuation, £60,000 for funeral, and £26,000 for accidents and other benefits.

Writing in 1898, Brabrook said that sick pay, superannuation, and funeral allowance, are benefits which can only be secured by the accumulation of considerable funds to meet the future accruing liability. But the members of trade unions, knowing what they want, disregard the teaching of the actuary. They do not accumulate large funds, nor do they earmark those funds for a special purpose. With an exception to which he refers there is not a single large trade union, says Brabrook at this time, which has as much as four years' income in hand; the average of all the unions is fifteen months' income only. The common practice is to levy each year as much as is required to meet the outgoings of the year and only to keep in hand a little over one year's income, except when the probability of a conflict is near, and it becomes necessary to increase the contributions of the members and accumulate a reserve to support them when the conflict comes. It is but justice to the trade unions to add that their members have made great sacrifices in order to keep faith with those to whom superannuation and other allowances have been promised.

We proceed to an examination of the four main types of friendlv society:—

(1) Accumulative Societies;

(2) Deposit Societies;

(3) Holloway Societies;

(4) Dividing Societies.

(1) *Accumulative Societies.*

These societies normally offer sickness and funeral benefits in return for a contribution which at the outset is designed to be sufficient to provide for them. Surplus is only appropriated on the basis of actuarial valuation, in which provision is made for the full liabilities, and the funds exist for the benefit of the society as a whole, except to the extent to which surplus may be allocated to members individually. The amount which a member may draw in sickness benefits depends upon the duration of his sickness, and his benefits do not cease merely because his own contributions may have been exhausted in sick pay received (although many societies impose a limit upon the total amount of sick pay receivable). In other words, in accumulative societies the true principle of insurance is in operation, combined with the recognition of actuarial principles.

The largest among the Accumulative Societies are the Affiliated Orders with their wide range of branches. There follow the centralised societies, the county societies and the large but rapidly diminishing number of small societies.[1] In the process of reduction in the small societies by amalgamation many have retained their separate identity.

The affiliated orders generally are of a triple formation; the basis is the Lodge, as it is called in the Oddfellows, the Court, in the Foresters, or the Tent, in the Rechabites. The lodge (court or tent) is the body which makes the primary contact with the member. Immediately above the lodge is the District. The District consists of the group of lodges in a particular area, and is governed by representatives from those lodges. Primarily the functions of the District are administrative. The lodge as a rule retains the sole responsibility

[1] In the course of the discussion on a paper read before the Institute of Actuaries in 1932, Mr. Epps said that there was a very great reduction in the number of sickness benefit societies, namely from three thousand to just over one thousand. This was largely due to the fact that by 1916 no less than sixteen hundred of them had dropped out, of which four hundred became branches of affiliated orders and probably got a new lease of life. It was no doubt the case that the decline was mainly due to the advent of the National Health Insurance scheme of 1912. Quite a number of capably managed societies with very considerable funds disappeared during the years immediately following. Generally they were societies which had not provided very large benefits, and when a large proportion of their members became subject to the National Health Insurance system had no desire to duplicate benefits and therefore were wound up.

for the sickness benefit; the District by a form of re-insurance assumes the liability for the death benefits or, as they are more commonly termed, funeral benefits. The chief financial function of the Order is to provide relief to those branches which fall into a condition of deficiency. The origin of district funeral funds is to be found chiefly in the realisation of the need for some connecting bond in the nature of a common interest between the lodges which would otherwise have been financially independent. With regard to the Order generally, the bonds of federation have usually been extraordinarily slight; there is no real chain to connect the various branches together and, unless some artificial one can be forged, such as a funeral fund or a relief fund, there is no basis for association beyond mere sentiment. Watson said, writing in 1912, that the most prominent work that the affiliated orders had undertaken during the preceding ten years had been a vigorous attempt to deal with deficiencies. In the best affiliated societies the valuations are followed by enquiry into joint measures of amelioration. In the Manchester Unity and in the Foresters there is a common recognition of the fact that when a sacrifice is demanded from the members to place themselves in a sound financial condition there must be a corresponding measure of assistance from the society at large. In the Manchester Unity it has been quite a common practice to require a reduction of sickness benefit or an increase of contribution and to take over the liability for part or the whole of the older members, e.g. the men over 60 years of age; if the whole liability in respect of such members is taken over, the district generally bears the cost of sickness benefit while the central body bears the charge for the death benefits.

After the Affiliated Orders the most important group is that of the centralized societies, of which the chief is the Hearts of Oak Benefit Society. In 1912 this society had a very large membership without any district branches or any other local or agency organization, the whole of the members sending their contributions quarterly by post to the central office. This system of sending contributions by post is one which distinguishes the centralized societies from the affiliated orders; apart from this it is perhaps unnecessary to say very much about the centralized societies. With regard to the Hearts of Oak Society it is observed from its annual reports that the policy and administration of this society is constantly reviewed in order to secure the greatest possible service to the membership. It was with this object in view that the system of local agencies was introduced in 1919. Since that date the great majority of the members, 92 per cent., have been brought within the scheme. The Hearts of Oak has also a board of delegates representing 226 districts, and the machinery therefore does not appear to be distinguishable in any material respect from that of collecting societies such as the Royal Liver and the Liverpool Victoria Societies.

The county societies form an interesting group; these were nearly always founded on strict actuarial principles, but most of them were established in the first half of the nineteenth century, and prior to 1911 remodelling of tables of experience had been necessary. In order to meet the growing sickness claims at the half-pay rate some of these societies had to reduce the benefit after a period to quarter-pay, and on this basis prosperity seems to have been assured. The societies of this class provide the opportunity of assuring deferred annuities. The contract for death benefit in these societies was separate from the sickness benefit.

(2) *Deposit Societies.*

The application of the insurance principle is, in greater or less degree, restricted by the system in operation in deposit societies. The member's contributions are not paid in their entirety into a common reserve and so made available for the payment of sickness benefits of all members alike, but are credited, either wholly or in part, to the member's individual account. When the member falls sick, a proportion of his sickness benefit is payable from his own account. The extent of this proportion—whether one-third, one-half, two-thirds, etc.—depends upon his age, occupation and state of health at entry, the contribution being normally the same for all ages at entry for the same total benefit. The balance of sickness benefit is payable either from the Common Sickness Fund, formed by the allocation of a fixed proportion of the contributions or from annual surplus income, or by a charge on the individual accounts of all the members. When a sick member has exhausted his own account, his right to claim upon the Common Sick Fund is restricted to the receipt of "grace pay" for a limited period, such right only being exercisable once in five years. A member may, however, when not sick, pay additional sums into his personal account and the ability to do this gives him an increased right to claim upon the Common Fund. One large society limits these payments to £30 in any calendar year, but there are wide differences of practice in this respect. At the end of each year (or other fixed period) the excess of the society's income over its expenditure, after providing for transfers to reserve funds, interest on members' deposit accounts, etc., is divided amongst the members and credited to their individual accounts.

There is a spirit of dissatisfaction among the old members, many of whom regularly paid their contributions for 20, 30, or 40 years, when they find that they stand no better in relation to the accumulated funds of that society than the young members who had recently joined. Watson says with regard to the deposit societies:

> "The keen desire of the members is to maintain their deposits, so that the system has a very pronounced effect in keeping down the claims. Whether it is quite right to minimise the claims with a possible hardship to the family of a member who from the state of his health would be better on the sick list is at least open to question. That is perhaps a point in sickness insurance morals that has not yet received the attention it deserves. The part of the common fund which is not drawn in sick pay during the year is divided up in proportion to the members' deposits at the end of the year. Members who are well-to-do need not limit their contributions; they can add to their deposits as much as they like. The result is that the members who are better off than the majority can add largely to their deposits and so get a title to obtain a great deal more from the common fund than the poorer members, although both classes are supposed to be paying on the same table of contribution. The system is thus subject to many contingencies, and it is not unfair to assume that the element of insurance is a secondary consideration with many of the contributors."

(3) *Holloway Societies.*

These societies, which are really a particular form of deposit societies, are based upon a system devised by Mr. George Holloway as operated in the Stroud Holloway Society founded by him in 1875.

One of the main principles governing their formation is that no benefit society can be considered as sound as it ought to be until it has established in its rules a principle for securing to every one of its members an annuity in old age. This is above all else the one thing needful.

The distinctive feature of this type of Society is that the contribution increases with the age of the member during the greater part of the period of his membership, and the annual contribution is fixed at an amount which is normally more than sufficient to cover the current cost of sickness claims. In the majority of these societies the contribution remains constant up to the age of 31 and then increases each year up to the age of 55 when it again becomes constant. Up to the age 45 or thereabouts the margin between the contribution available for sickness benefits and the current sickness risk is actually increased, and then it begins to diminish until it may even disappear altogether as the member approaches age 65, when membership usually terminates. In some cases where membership continues up to age 70, the sickness cost for the last few years may be in excess of the contribution received. At the end of each year the "profits" of the society, i.e., the excess of the income over the expenditure, are divided amongst the members and credited to their individual accounts, such accounts being entitled to interest year by year. On the attainment of the age at which sickness benefits cease, the member is entitled to withdraw the amount standing to his credit or to invest it in the purchase of an annuity. Should the member die before reaching that age the amount of his deposit is payable as death benefit and sometimes there is a guaranteed minimum payment on death.

The obvious defect of the Holloway system is the inequity which results from the allocation of an equal dividend to all members irrespective of age, seeing that the amounts contributed by them to the profit may vary very considerably and even become a negative quantity. Moreover, until the society has reached the condition of a stationary population, it depends for the maintenance of its dividend upon its ability to secure new members in progressively increasing numbers.

(4) *Dividing Societies.*

These societies do not provide for increasing contributions according to attained age and more often than not the contributions are not even graduated according to age at entry. The annual surplus of income over expenditure, usually after providing for a reserve fund on some "rule of thumb" basis, is distributed in cash to the members. The amount of funds retained in hand by these societies varies considerably. In approximately 40 per cent. of them the funds represent less than 10s. per member, but in a small minority they may amount to as much as £10 per member or even more. The difficulty which dividing societies experience is that they are dependent upon the accession of new members for the maintenance of the cash dividend, and unless these can be persuaded to join the dividend diminishes thereby further reducing the attractiveness of the society and accelerating its inevitable end.

One may quote Brabrook's sentiments without agreeing with his sweeping generalisations:

> "It seems a common mistake," he says, "on the part of legislators that it is within their province to find out for the people that which is for their good and that which is not, to encourage them to follow the former, and to devise brave punishments for those who will persist in following the latter. This is an absolute error: the province of the legislature is to find out what contracts people desire to enter into, and, when they have entered into them, to see that they fulfil them; not to tell them what contracts they ought to enter into, and what contracts they ought not to enter into. The administrators of the law may not be going beyond their province in offering such advice and guidance as experience may have shown to be useful; but, in general, people are the best judges of their own affairs, and know their own interests better than the wisest statesman who ever made a blunder—and no statesman ever did anything who did not do that. Hence the circumstance that Dividing Societies are popular leads to the conclusion that it is not without reason that they are so. They possess the advantage, that, as a member gets back his surplus payments at the end of the year, he is willing to pay more than the member of a society which looks forward only to the dim and distant future. They also have this advantage, that they frankly provide only for such sickness and death as may occur in the course of the current year. There is no affectation of providing for old age, either directly or indirectly."

With the tendency shewn by a number of accumulating societies to modify their system in favour of deposit or dividing methods, it seems desirable to examine a little more closely the methods of deposit and dividing societies and the extent of the security offered by them for their members' benefit. Deposit and dividing societies have one feature in common—they each aim at returning to the members periodically in whole or in part the excess of the societies' income over its expenditure—the one as a credit to his individual account, the other as an immediate dividend.

Sickness has usually been the main contingency against which friendly societies have striven to provide, and many of the earlier societies came to an end because they failed to recognise the fact that the liability for sickness increases as the age of the member advances, and made insufficient provision for the increased burden on the societies' funds which thus arises. Much of the earlier friendly society legislation was designed to encourage the formation of societies on a secure basis, but for many years it was hampered by the lack of information necessary to forecast with any accuracy the liabilities which a society would incur as its members grew older. The earlier Friendly Societies Acts were mainly concerned to encourage only societies formed on a sound basis, and at one stage, as we have already noted, the Act required that, before a friendly society could enjoy the advantages conferred by it, the tables adopted must be certified by an actuary employed by an insurance company. But from 1875 onwards legislation permitted societies to be registered without regard to their soundness, and required instead that they should be periodically valued with a view to discovering the sufficiency, or otherwise, of the reserves which they had accumulated.

Many of the existing deposit and dividing societies have introduced expedients of various kinds to make some provision for a future increase in their liabilities. In some instances the provision may give the society a large measure of security. Circumstances change, however, and unless the financial position of a society is periodically tested, as it is for an accumulating society by valuation, there is no guarantee that the expedient adopted will be adequate for future security.

In the case of a dividing society in which the contracts terminate at the end of each year no question of valuation arises, although even in such cases the guidance of an actuary would seem to be desirable in the process of fixing the scale of contributions to be charged, or the amount of the reserve which it is desirable to retain in hand.

This is in substance what Watson said some years ago, and I

think it desirable to append a note here of what may be achieved in the case of a dividing society which submits to valuation. The following extract from a letter which I have received from Mr. Rockliff with regard to his own society, The New Tabernacle Approved Society, is of interest in this connection.

> "When I founded the New Tabernacle Dividing Society, now 50 years ago, I expressly stated that it should be regarded by its members as supplementary to and not in substitution for a more permanent benefit provision. Nevertheless I directed my efforts, in relation to its financial basis, towards making it an ideal dividing society, after which other similar societies might strive. Thus, I never divided the funeral fund. I paid a fixed dividend of a lesser sum than was possible, and built up a reserve with the balance.
>
> "My successor, some six years ago, felt justified in describing the dividend, not as 'fixed' (my own term), but as 'guaranteed.' This caught the eye of the late Government Actuary and he persuaded the Chief Registrar to call upon the Society to submit to actuarial valuation. This was in due course undertaken. The Funeral Fund of £107,000 was found to be in surplus, and the Sickness Fund (after allowing for an annual return of the fixed dividend out of surplus contributions) showed a solvency of 18s. 8d. in the £, which would be turned into 20s. in the £ by the stoppage of benefit and contributions when the pension age of 65 was reached. At present there is no such limit. The Valuation Report has been submitted by the Registry of Friendly Societies to the Treasury, and the Society has now been told that the dividend is as near to 'guaranteed' as makes no odds."

A scheme which possesses features of unusual interest is that of the Mutual Thrift Tables of the Hearts of Oak Benefit Society. The membership under these tables, which were prepared under actuarial guidance, is divided into four sections:—

(a) Males following non-hazardous occupations.

(b) Males following hazardous occupations (Two sections).

(c) Females.

The contributions, which are graduated according to age at entry, include, for each section, an amount transferable to the member's "Personal Thrift Account." The portion of the contribution available for sickness benefits is treated differently according as the member elects to join one or other of the two divisions into which each section is divided.

If the member joins the "Individual Account Section," one-half of his sickness benefit is payable from his own personal account, built up by the transfer thereto of one-half of his sickness contributions, and this half ceases when his account is exhausted. The other half of his sickness benefit is payable, as long as sickness continues, from the "Common Sick Fund." In this way the member secures something of the advantages of the deposit system without its disadvantages, as the sickness benefit is permanent to the extent of one-half. Members who have not elected to join this section receive the whole of their benefit from the "Common Sick Fund."

The "Personal Thrift Accounts" and "Individual Sickness Accounts" are credited annually with interest, whilst the former receive a share of any surplus disclosed by the annual actuarial valuations of the "Common Sick Fund."

The valuation of the Thrift Tables tends to show that the members who join the Individual Account Section experience lighter rates of sickness than members who draw the whole of their benefit from the Common Sick Fund.

Under the stress of competition from the Holloway and deposit societies, many of the accumulative societies (as noted at the end of the previous chapter) have adopted schemes which offer benefits on somewhat similar lines. A number of societies—particularly county—have for very many years past met the demand for the deposit society type of benefit by creating a separate deposit or Holloway section. More recently, however, a number of schemes have been adopted which involve no departure from sound actuarial principles. The main feature of these schemes is the addition to an ordinary sickness contract providing for sickness benefits up to the age of 65 or 70 of a contribution which is accumulated at a fixed rate of interest so as to yield a lump sum payment on the attainment of the age of 65. In the event of death before that age the accumulated amount of the supplementary contributions is payable with a guaranteed minimum, smaller sums being payable on withdrawal.

I have not thought it necessary to describe in this section the constitution of Collecting Societies and Industrial Insurance Companies, which play such a considerable part in the National Health Insurance scheme, as their constitution and machinery, in broad outline, are really matters of common knowledge ; reference is made elsewhere to their general administration.

This account of the activities of the societies which became the approved societies under the National Health Insurance Scheme may be conveniently concluded with a summary of the position under that scheme at the time of the Report of the Royal Commission on National Health Insurance (as given at page 10 of the Report).

"There are at the present time about 1,000 Approved Societies engaged in the administration of the Act, including 31 Societies with Branches. The Branches, which number about 7,000, are independent financial units for the purpose of National Health Insurance; they possess also a considerable measure of administrative independence, but are integral parts of the parent organisations to which respectively they belong and are subject to the general authority thereof. Approved Societies are not as a rule organised on any territorial basis, though in the nature of the case the membership of many of them is preponderantly localised. They vary in membership from less than 50 to more than 2,000,000 insured persons. Some are restricted to persons engaged in particular occupations or belonging to particular religious denominations or having some other common bond of interest; while others are open to all insured persons without qualification. For certain purposes Approved Societies may also be conveniently viewed in relation to other work carried on by them or their promoters, and from this point of view they may be classified into societies formed in the Friendly Society movement, those instituted by the great Industrial Insurance Companies, those organised in connection with Trade Unions, and various other types of less importance numerically. Of these latter societies promoted by employers may be cited as a group which presents features distinguishing them in certain respects from other societies. This division of the insured population into self-contained units is a fundamental feature of the present Scheme and it leads to remarkable consequences, both of a financial and of a social nature. The surpluses built up vary over a very wide range owing to the diversity of sickness and maternity experience in the different societies, and the scales of additional benefits which can be provided are correspondingly varied."

(b) *Effects on Membership and Funds.*

I propose in this section to give statements which I have obtained from the secretaries of some of the largest societies setting out the growth of membership and funds of these societies, with additional notes which may be of interest in this connection.

Tabular statements, with notes, are furnished, setting out particulars of the membership and funds for the parent or voluntary societies as distinct from those administering the National Health Insurance scheme. The numbers of the Approved Societies valued and the membership of those societies as at the different valuations is given also in a tabular statement compiled from the Government Actuary's reports. The actual results of the valuations, with particulars of surpluses disclosed on valuation, are reserved for a later chapter.

Before giving these particulars it is necessary to make a brief statement concerning the operation of section 72 of the National Health Insurance Act, 1911. This was a section from which the members of the old friendly societies had been led to expect great things. It gave an enormous amount of work and in the result very little was done. The principal part of the section is as follows: —

> "Every registered friendly society which provides benefits similar to any of those conferred by this Part of this Act, shall submit to the Registrar of Friendly Societies a scheme for continuing, abolishing, reducing, or altering such benefits as respects members who become insured persons and for continuing, abolishing, or reducing the contributions of such members, so, however, that the combined effect of the alteration of the benefits and contributions shall not prejudicially affect the solvency of the society."

Watson, in his sixth lecture published in the book "Friendly Society Finance" to which I have already given a reference, says with regard to this section, "It expresses the idea that, with 10s. per week insured to him as sick pay from the State scheme, it is no longer necessary for the member to insure the full benefits from his society for which he had subscribed previously, and that, correspondingly with the responsibility placed on him of paying 4d. a week to the State scheme there ought to be some measure of release from the contributions which he has contracted to pay to his society. That, obviously, is a reasonable proposition."

Watson also points out that " the section does not give to the member whose contract is readjusted the exact value of the amount of liability of which the society is set free in his case. It throws the amount released into a general pool to be dealt with, if the society chooses, as a whole, and does not give any individual the right to claim that the difference between his full reserve value and his reduced reserve value shall be dealt with as a sum available for his own particular use."

I have not been able to obtain very much information as to the extent to which societies or branches submitted schemes for reducing benefit and contributions, but there appears to be general agreement that the number was relatively small and that the financial factor in such reductions as took place was of very little significance. It was nothing approaching that which was anticipated though, obviously, to the extent to which reserves were released which had been held on behalf of members of a society, the operation strengthened that society financially to a limited extent. It is worth noting that some of the members who reduced their payments found themselves in difficulty at age 70 when they were required to go back to their original contribution; at that age they became entitled to their original rate of sickness benefit from the independent society despite anything they might receive under the Old Age Pension Acts, either contributory or non-contributory.

As very little use was made of section 72 by members of societies for reducing their former provision it may be inferred that in the majority of cases the members who had formerly made provision for benefits comparable with those under the National Health Insurance Act continued their contribution at the old rate and were, therefore, insured for these sums in supplementation of the benefits provided under the National Health Insurance scheme. It will be clear in the statements which follow how the ordinary wastage of members of the old types of friendly society has not been completely made good, and that the trend of membership in the case of those coming under the National Health Insurance scheme for the first time has been entirely on the side of the Collecting and Industrial Assurance Companies and the Deposit Friendly Societies. If there is anyone at this date who is sufficiently interested to learn more about section 72, he would do well to read Watson's sixth lecture, to which I have referred.

One of the early changes in benefit arrangements effected by many friendly societies after the passing of the National Insurance Act 1911 was the adoption of tables for new entrants which provided for the cessation of sickness benefits at age 70. The need for action in this direction arose somewhat earlier than 1911 owing to the passing of the Old Age Pensions Act in 1908, but the provision of sickness benefit ceasing at age 70 under the State scheme served to focus the problem more clearly and rendered easier the passing of the necessary reforms. It will be readily understood that the receipt of a pension concurrently with sickness benefit is likely to lead to an increase in the claims for the latter benefit, and it was the realisation of this fact, and the recognition by those responsible for administering sickness benefits of the great difficulty of distinguishing between disability resulting merely from old age and that due to a specific ailment, that led most of the affiliated orders and of the other larger societies to adopt, in 1912 or thereabouts, tables for new entrants which provided for the cessation of sickness benefits at age 70, with or without an annuity benefit thereafter.

The passing of the Widows', Orphans' and Old Age Contributory Pensions Acts 1925, which provided for the grant of pensions at age 65 for a much larger section of the population than would have satisfied the means qualification of the original Act, has rendered the solution of the problem of excessive rates of sickness at the older ages still more urgent. It is obvious that as far as new members are concerned the proper course is to adopt new tables granting sickness benefits ceasing at age 65, but societies have been very hesitant to take this step. Many of them exhibit an unwillingness to invite new members to join on the basis of a sickness benefit ceasing at age 65 which is not followed by an annuity, but they also maintain that the cost of the combined benefit is so heavy that it is not possible to secure new members upon such a basis. Even if societies were all to adopt for new entrants tables providing sickness benefits ceasing at age 65, they would still be left with the problem of the probable increase in claims after that age in respect of existing members assured for sickness benefits throughout life or to the age of 70. Some few societies have substituted for sick pay after age 70 an annuity of equivalent value, but owing to the smallness of the annuity which can be allowed this solution has not proved to be popular. Where a society possesses a considerable surplus and the rate of reduced sick pay does not fall below one-half of full pay, it is sometimes practicable to apply the surplus in producing an annuity which the members are prepared to accept in commutation of sick pay, but it is unlikely that more than a small minority of societies can be persuaded to adopt this plan. The need to fix the commutation age at 65 instead of 70 reduces still further the attractiveness of the equivalent annuity.

An alternative method which it has been found possible to adopt in some few cases provides for the grant of an endowment at age 65 or 70, in lieu of future sickness benefit. But so far no really satisfactory scheme capable of general application has been devised for relieving societies of the heavy additional liability which appears likely to fall upon them in respect of members insured for sickness benefits beyond the age of 65.

The figures extracted from the reports and returns supplied to me by secretaries of several large societies are now set out, followed by Statement A prepared by the Chief Registrar; with full notes appended of the general conclusions to be drawn from the Statement.

No particular purpose is to be served by an examination of the Prudential figures as distinct from the summarised returns for Collecting Societies and Industrial Assurance Companies, of which the Prudential Society forms so substantial a part.

Independent Order of Oddfellows
Manchester Unity.

Number of adult members :

Year	1909	883,000
	1914	989,000
	1936	901,000

VALUATIONS.

Date.	Present Value of Benefits Assured.	Present Value of Assets applicable thereto.	Net Deficiencies.	Net Surplus.
	£	£	£	£
1904-7	24,117,000	24,525,000	—	408,000
*1911	25,657,000	25,624,000	33,000	—
†1925-1927	25,211,000	28,651,000	—	3,440,000
‡1930-1933	26,922,000	29,217,000	—	2,295,000

* On this occasion the basis of the Valuations was changed to the 1893-1897 Experience.

† This is the first valuation based upon the original benefits and contributions in respect of the whole of the membership.

‡ The basis of this valuation was appreciably stronger than that of the preceding valuations.

The following statement with regard to the Manchester Unity is of interest:—

Extract from the Report of the Chief Registrar of Friendly Societies for the year 1929.

The report of the actuaries on the twelfth valuation of the Independent Order of Oddfellows, Manchester Unity, is now available. In this Order the total surpluses amounted to £3,669,000 and deficiencies to £229,000, making a net surplus of £3,440,000 in respect of benefits valued at £25,211,000. As compared with the eleventh valuation of the Order the balance of surplus has increased by about £700,000 despite the fact that in many lodges benefits have been increased or contributions reduced in order to restore scales which had previously been in force. The operation of restoring such scales may now be said to have been brought to a successful conclusion, and on the success of the operation the Order is entitled to congratulation. The Order as a whole is in a strong position financially without any sacrifice of the benefits originally promised to the members.

Sickness experience, although on the whole lighter than the experience of 1893-97 assumed in the valuation, shows an increase over the experience disclosed in the eleventh valuation. The mortality experience was as a whole only 76 per cent. of that expected under the tables used, which results in a strain on the sickness and superannuation funds. The valuers state that fortunately the existence in the case of most lodges of a fairly considerable margin between the rate of interest earned upon the funds and the rate assumed in the valuation has so far yielded profits sufficient to meet the additional strain, but that the limit of the improvement in vitality has certainly not been reached, and it will be necessary to make specific provision for it in the next valuation.

Ancient Order of Foresters.

Membership at the end of 1910	760,000
,, ,, ,, 1936	725,000
Funds in 1910	£9,375,000
,, 1936	£17,731,000

The valuations show the greatly strengthened position of the Order, a net deficit of nearly £2,500,000 in 1896 having been converted into a net surplus approaching £1,500,000 in 1932—and this, notwithstanding the fact that the basis of valuation had become more stringent, the post-war valuations having been made upon Watson's tables, M.U. experience 1893-7, with appropriate loadings where necessary.

Hearts of Oak Benefit Society.

Membership and Funds :

Year.	No. of Members.	Amount of Reserve Funds.
1912	567,000	£4,252,000
1922	595,000	£6,372,000
1932	734,000	£9,783,000
1936	806,000	£11,867,000

When the National Health Insurance Act became operative in 1912 the original group was closed to new entrants and six new Tables were formed. During the year 1919 further Tables of membership were formed, and from time to time since, including the Society's Thrift Tables, the membership of which now exceeds 100,000.

Broadway Congregational Friendly Society.

The following figures of membership are those of a predominantly local society with only a very small membership before the N.H.I. scheme. The parent society was founded by the deacons of the church for the service of those whose voluntary contributions could be brought to Hammersmith Broadway. The society has no branches or agents.

Year.	Voluntary Membership.	State Membership.
1910	725	nil
1913	1,460	3,000
1937	16,388	9,437

THE NATIONAL DEPOSIT FRIENDLY SOCIETY.

The growth of this society from the year 1888 when it had 6,536 members and £28,000 funds is the most remarkable in the whole Friendly Society movement outside the Collecting Societies which are grouped for the purpose of this review with the Industrial Assurance Companies.

Here are a few figures of the Deposit section. The membership of the State section at the end of 1936 was approximately 723,000.

Year	Members	Funds
		£
1908	185,000	947,000
1918	456,000	2,710,000
1930	1,040,000	7,666,000
1936	1,368,000	11,485,000

THE NEW TABERNACLE SICK AND PROVIDENT SOCIETY.

In the case of a Dividing Society it is necessary to look at the sums paid in benefits and bonuses to measure the progress, but this particular dividing society had a Funeral Fund Reserve of £107,000 at the end of 1937 (reference is made to this earlier in the chapter). The record of membership etc. is as follows.

Year.	Membership.	Sick Pay	Funeral Benefit.	Bonus.
		£	£	£
1911	10,300	3,600	800	14,000
1937	23,000	13,800	4,500	31,000

The growth of the sick-pay relatively to the membership is noteworthy; the bonus (the "share-out" at Christmas) is the principal benefit.

THE HOLLOWAY GROUP.

The membership return of the National Union of Holloway Friendly Societies comprising some 30 societies, of which the largest is the Ideal Benefit Society (Birmingham), gives the following figures for 1936.

	Private Side.	State Side.
Male members	406,000	269,000
Female ,,	75,000	107,000

The numbers included in these totals for the Ideal Benefit Society are. –

Male members	94,000	95,000
Female ,,	17,000	43,000

I have not the comparative figures for an earlier year except in the case of the Stroud Holloway Original Benefit Society, started by the founder of the movement.

The figures are as follows:—

	Membership.	Funds.
		£
Year 1911	5,589	133,000
1937	13,604	397,000

COLLECTING SOCIETIES AND INDUSTRIAL ASSURANCE COMPANIES.

When we turn to examine the returns of the societies in this group, figures of "Membership" except in the "Approved Society" section are rather meaningless and the figures are therefore given showing the growth of funds in the parent society and the membership of the Approved Society. The question of surpluses and valuation results is not examined in this paper in the case of any particular society, but is dealt with elsewhere in groups.

ROYAL LIVER FRIENDLY SOCIETY ACCUMULATED FUNDS.

1910	..	..	£3,386,000
1915	..	..	4,290,000
1925	..	..	10,717,000
1937	..	..	24,950,000

The membership of the National Health section in 1912 was 326,000 in the proportion of 8 men to 5 women; at the end of 1933, the membership was 486,000, in, roughly, the same proportion.

Industrial Assurance Premium Income and Funds of the Parent Bodies of the National Amalgamated Approved Society.

Year.	Industrial Assurance Premium Income.	Industrial Assurance Funds.
	£	£
1910	7,106,000	11,145,000
1915	8,479,000	15,777,000
1925	16,753,000	47,589,000
1935	23,796,000	105,291,000

Membership of the National Amalgamated Approved Society.

Year.	Membership (approx.)
1913	1,907,000
1933	2,605,000

In the statement which is subjoined figures of membership and benefits are given for all types of societies for the years 1910 and 1934.

FRIENDLY SOCIETIES.

(Statement A)

COMPARISON OF FIGURES FOR 1910 WITH 1934.

	Adult Membership		Benefits						Funds	
			Sickness		Death		Other			
	1910 £ 000's	1934 £ 000's	1910 £ 000's	1934 £ 000's	1910 £ 000's	1934 £ 000's	1910 £ 000's	1934 £ 000's	1910 £ 000's	1934 £ 000's
Societies without branches :—										
Societies providing sickness benefits (with or without other benefits) :—										
Accumulating	1,314	1,144	1,178	1,250	215	358	317	1,058	13,482	33,537
Deposit	381	1,912	164	981	16	155	230	1,368	3,498	22,614
Dividing	245	409	91	271	31	105	239	500	294	879
Burial & W. & O.	1,012	347	—	—	120	73	104	110	2,923	2,991
Medical	329	143	—	—	—	—	57	136	64	191
Societies providing annuities, pensions, endowments and miscellaneous benefits ..	440	811	—	—	18	123	312	1,075	1,699	17,649
Orders and Branches	3,721	4,766	1,433	2,502	400	814	1,259	4,247	21,960	77,861
	2,783*	2,918*	2,197	2,646	487	636	419	Not available	27,934	52,052
Total	6,504	7,684	3,630	5,148	887	1,450	1,678		49,894	129,913

*Includes juveniles—both years.

INDUSTRIAL ASSURANCE.

	No. of Policies		Funds	
	1913 000's	1934 000's	1913 000's	1934 000's
Collecting Societies	7,481	21,752	11,165	65,720
Companies	37,556	68,324	55,762	277,518
Total	45,037	90,076	£66,927	£343,238

Examination of the figures set out in Statement A shows that the membership of all centralized Friendly Societies and Orders combined has been more than maintained; there is an actual increase of one-sixth or more than one million persons. This figure of increase, however, is a balance of losses and gains. On the one hand, the accumulative societies, i.e., those insuring against sickness on an accumulative basis show the following losses of membership:—

(*a*) The centralized societies, excluding Juvenile societies, a loss of 170,000 on the pre-war figure of 1,300,000.

(*b*) The Orders and Branches show a slight gain on the 1910 figure, but this gain is more than wiped out by the loss sustained by the "accumulating" (centralized) societies. (The gain in the case of the Orders is due wholly to increased juvenile membership; it is also necessary to bear in mind that there has been a partial centralization of benefits adopted in some Orders, and also some development of the individual account and deposit systems.)

Further losses of members are to be noted in the case of societies insuring against death, but not sickness. These show a reduction of some ¾-million, mainly due to the fact that some of the old Burial Societies employing collectors are now merged in the Collecting Societies, with the figures included under Industrial Assurance, and no longer appear as Friendly Society business. The membership of Medical Societies shows a loss of some 185,000, a diminution of about 60 per cent.

Where there are gains in Friendly Society membership, the figures are somewhat spectacular. There are three groups, (1) Deposit, (2) Dividing, and (3) Miscellaneous Societies providing mainly for old age, (viz. pension, annuity and endowment assurance), which may be referred to as "Old Age" Societies. The group also includes Societies for institutional treatment in sickness or convalescence, and also Miners Accident Societies, but the bulk of the increase is of the "Old Age" type. These three classes have more than made good the losses which have been referred to, and consequently the Friendly Societies as a whole show substantial gains in membership.

(1) The Deposit Societies; the increase is five-fold, the numbers being under 400,000 in 1910, and now nearly 2,000,000.

(2) Dividing Societies show a gain of 164,000 on a pre-war figure of 245,000.

(3) The miscellaneous societies with a pre-war figure of 440,000 have very nearly doubled their membership.

When we turn to the figures for the Industrial Assurance group, the increases shown in the aggregate numbers in the Friendly Society group fade into insignificance. The number of policies effected with Collecting Societies and Industrial Assurance Companies show an increase of 100 per cent., the growth being from 45,000,000 to 90,000,000. (These figures can only be explained in relation to population, by the fact that numbers of separate assurances are frequently effected on the life of one person). In the total increase under this head it will be observed that the number of policies of Collecting Societies has grown from 7,500,000 to 21,500,000, and of the Industrial Assurance Companies from 37,500,000 to 68,500,000.

The growth of funds has out-stripped the growth of membership at every point, the Friendly Societies showing a 160 per cent. increase on the 1910 total of £50,000,000. The Funds of the Collecting Societies have grown from £11,000,000 to £65,000,000, and those of the Industrial Assurance Companies from 56,000,000 to 277,000,000.

The following general conclusions may be drawn from the examination of the statement:—

(1) Since the advent of National Health Insurance the "voluntary" funds of the Industrial Assurance and Friendly Society groups, taken together, show an expansion equivalent in amount to more than double the present Health and Pension Funds under the State scheme, and are not far short of the total capital invested in Building Societies.

(2) There has been a remarkable movement of Friendly Society insurance towards provision of some kind for old age, even in the ordinary Friendly Societies. There is a trend in the direction of substitution of small pension for sickness benefit, at the age when the member also becomes eligible for State pension.

The other two major features are those to which attention has already been drawn. (3) The increasingly successful competition of Deposit and Dividing Societies in the sphere of Sickness insurance with societies of the accumulative type, and (4) in the case of Death Benefit and Endowment Assurance, the astonishingly rapid progress made by companies and societies employing collectors.

There is no doubt that the outlook of friendly society members is undergoing a marked change—their attitude towards societies is more individualistic than formerly. New entrants are much more prone to view membership in the light of a business contract from which they will endeavour to obtain the maximum advantage for themselves. The appeal which was successful in the past in obtaining members, viz., association, with the object of mutual sharing of burdens, now usually falls on deaf ears; the prospective member is more anxious about benefits that he will himself enjoy, and he is not content to know merely what he will get if he is sick and what benefit at death, but asks what he will get out of the society if he is not sick and survives to a ripe age or if he should desire to leave the society. The ordinary friendly society is handicapped in obtaining new entrants from young people who view things from this angle if the society continues to offer only types of assurance which have made it successful in the past, viz., maximum sickness and death benefits obtainable with security relatively to such contribution as the member can afford to pay. Deposit societies can point to members' individual accounts which accumulate for old age or are withdrawable earlier subject only to some forfeiture. Dividing societies can point to their dividends. Industrial assurance companies substitute endowment assurance for whole life policies and point to free policies and surrender values.

Friendly societies complain strongly about industrial assurance competition and the part it plays in National Health Insurance—some even have themselves become collecting societies to compete with the companies and older collecting societies which are successfully building up new business, not, it is fairly argued, because they can be conducted more cheaply, but by reason of the access their paid representatives have to homes of the people.

However efficiently conducted, house to house collection of contributions is necessarily costly, and while it would be a great pity if friendly societies generally resort to this system to maintain membership they may ask: if they do not, what attractions can they add to their benefits to enable them to withstand more successfully keen competition?

Whether Deposit and Dividing systems will prove as successful as in the past now that they are being required to submit to the test of valuation is a question not yet determined. Anyway, the older types of societies must absorb the moral that there is nothing inherently wrong in these newer systems, provided sufficient reserves are accumulated and maintained so as to place the societies on a solvent and permanent footing.

The older type of friendly society offers no compensation to a member who for any reason is unable to continue membership, while organisations which are competing successfully do—the Deposit society adds the attraction of what appears to be a double barreled benefit, one that will serve either as a provision against death during that period of a member's life when it is most needed, or, if he survives beyond that period, can be switched over to serve as some provision for old age. The Dividing society is attractive in spite of the short period for which sickness benefit can usually be claimed, because the member is persuaded that he recovers any surplus on his insurance at a time when he can make good use of it, instead of storing it up in the society. One attraction of industrial assurance is the right to free policy or surrender value imposed by law. The companies have not been slow to see the advantages of this from a competitive standpoint—in some instances they go beyond what is required of them by statute. Policy-holders also have a statutory right to refer disputes to a commissioner, and the commissioner has the power in certain conditions of appointing an inspector without application from policy-holders.

Other directions in which the industrial assurance undertakings can claim an advantage over friendly societies is in the greater security offered against insolvency—they may be wound up compulsorily if they fail to maintain solvency, and in the protection to some extent against dishonest officials through compulsory audit by public auditors. Needless to say these undertakings make the most of these advantages in canvassing members. The assurance companies also have a greater scope in that they can assure a wider range of relations.

Amongst inducements which might make for success in obtaining members, the older societies might explore the following:

(1) A "surplus" contribution recoverable as a periodical cash distribution, or accumulated for old age, or earlier withdrawal

subject to some penalty. This need not be a distribution fixed in amount per member, and might vary with the fortunes of the society if provision for accumulation of reserves is fixed by the valuer for the period ensuing till next valuation.

(2) Some concession in the way of surrender value on lapsing in certain circumstances, with an alternative of reduced benefit free of future contributions..

(3) Some form of death benefit exchangeable in later life for a pension for rest of life.

(4) Better benefits for juveniles, including more generous bonus allowances on transfer to adult societies.

Industrial assurance undertakings are also developing reversionary and cash bonuses as an added attraction—in some sense analogous to accumulations in members' individual accounts and periodical cash dividends in Deposit and Dividing societies. Obviously all these additional attractions of supplementary and more elastic benefits must come out of the members' pockets in some fashion as an added margin of contribution.

There is one direction in which National Health Insurance has left a gap which friendly societies might be expected to fill—provision for sickness in that section of the community not in insurable employment but nevertheless in need of some provision; this includes the large and important class of wives not in paid employment and children under age of entry into employment. There is, of course, a serious risk in extending ordinary sickness benefit in this direction. It is a sound principle of insurance that the insured ought not to benefit financially by the occurrence of the contingency insured against; normally wives and children are not wage-earners and provision of sickness benefit for them would mean that sickness would bring money into the home. Provision of medical aid, home nursing and institutional care on a much better footing might, however, be considered; so long as the benefit is provided in kind, there is no inducement to claim except in real need.

Instead of considering switching over to other systems, as some of the older friendly societies are already commencing to do, they might be well advised to consider first whether their existing systems cannot be modified to confer advantages equivalent to those which attract members elsewhere, in such manner as to avoid sacrifice of the principles which have served them so well in the past.

As it would be of interest to give a full statement as to the growth of the business of Industrial Assurance, I have set out in Appendix No. 2 a statement showing the growth of business amongst Industrial Assurance Companies and Collecting Societies between the years 1877 and 1936, the figures for the last twenty years having been taken from the Industrial Assurance Commissioner's annual reports. In the same appendix figures with regard to the growth of whole life and endowment assurance are given for the years 1925, 1930 and 1935, these figures having also been extracted from the reports of the Industrial Assurance Commissioner.

In order that the statistics of membership and funds of the whole of the groups which constitute the registered provident societies may be seen in relation to one another, I have extracted the information set out in Appendix No. 3.

Concurrently with the period of development of National Health Insurance, and largely, it may fairly be claimed, with the educational value of experience gained in the administration of the national scheme, there has been a remarkable improvement in the soundness of the whole friendly society movement. I have made an examination of the whole series of Reports of the Chief Registrar of Friendly Societies and I give the following extracts from 1924 onwards; they are reassuring and speak for themselves.

Extract from the Report of the Chief Registrar of Friendly Societies for the Year 1924.

The total surpluses exceed the total deficiencies. This is probably the first period in which this has occurred during the long history of the Friendly Society movement.

The valuations included in the period of one year covered by this report shows surpluses amounting to £7,523,000 and deficiencies of £6,481,000, whereas the corresponding figures for the previous valuations of the same societies were £4,812,000 and £11,110,000 respectively. So that the increase in the total surpluses added to the reduction in the total deficiencies amounts to a sum of no less than £7,340,000.

Extract for the Year 1925.

There have been very large reductions in deficiencies resulting from alterations in the benefits or contributions. There is clear evidence that officials of societies are becoming increasingly alive to the importance of dealing with valuation deficiencies as soon as they are disclosed. In most of the larger societies with branches the rules contain provisions requiring branches with deficiencies to make such alterations in the contracts of the members as will bring the degree of solvency up to a certain minimum. In a number of the large Orders there exists a central fund, derived from a levy on the surpluses of solvent branches, or by direct contributions from all the branches, for assisting those in an insolvent position. The financial effect of such rules has been very considerable. It has been supplemented by the efforts made by the Chief Registrar to induce insolvent societies and branches to undertake measures of reform, efforts which, it is satisfactory to note, have met with considerable success. Although it has not always been possible to persuade the members to take such measures as will entirely remove the deficiency, it is only in a comparatively few cases that they refuse to take any steps at all. The difficulties that confront the officials of societies with substantial deficiencies are fully appreciated. The increase in contributions or reduction in benefits necessary to restore solvency may be so considerable that to carry them out in their entirety is impracticable. In such circumstances it is suggested that consideration should be given to the question of making the contributions and sickness benefits cease at age 65, at which age the majority of the members will presumably become entitled, after 1st January, 1928, to pensions under the Widows' Orphans' and Old Age Contributory Pensions Act of 1925. This alteration would greatly improve the financial position, in many cases resulting in complete solvency. The difficulties of administering sickness benefit in the case of members in receipt of old age pensions are known, and will, presumably, be increased with the reduction of the pension age to 65.

Extract for the Year 1926.

In both societies without branches and societies with branches the figures in the table show further increases in total surplus and decrease in total deficiency. Both types of society now show in the aggregate an excess of assets over liabilities—in the case of societies without branches for the first time. In regard to the societies without branches the figures are remarkable, the increase in surpluses amounting to nearly £500,000, while there is a decrease of over £50,000 in the deficiencies in spite of a deficiency of over £200,000 in the first valuation of a pension society. The net improvement has thus amounted to over £550,000, as compared with an improvement of £375,000 in 1925 and a deterioration of £1,000 in 1924. The extent of any progress indicated by the figures from year to year is necessarily affected by the size and number of valuations which fall into a particular year. The distribution is uneven, and the comparatively large improvement shown in the figures received in 1926 is due mainly to the fact that during that year the proportion of large societies re-valued was exceptionally high. The societies insuring benefits during sickness still show a balance of deficiency, but even this has been considerably reduced. It is satisfactory to note that the improvement in the financial position, although in some cases due to reductions of benefits or increases of contributions, in the majority of the societies, has been brought about by lighter rates of sickness claims and more profitable investment of the funds, which have not only resulted in substantial profits to the societies concerned but have rendered justifiable less stringent bases of valuation.

The question of dealing with deficiencies disclosed by valuation has been referred to at some length in recent reports, but there is one point which often seems to be overlooked when proposals for remedying them are under consideration. To remove any considerable deficiency it is generally necessary to modify the contributions or benefits, or both, but it does not follow that these alterations should apply to new entrants. In many such cases the contributions are sufficient to provide the benefits to new members, and it is clearly inequitable that they should be called upon to bear the burden of a deficiency for which they are in no way responsible. Nor is the society likely to induce any substantial number of persons to join it if the contributions and benefits to be paid in respect of new entrants compare unfavourably with those of other societies.

There have been cases where, in response to an enquiry as to what steps are to be taken to reduce the deficiency, the society has intimated that it was hoped to improve matters by enrolling new members. Such a proceeding cannot be too strongly reprobated. In effect it is proposed to make good the shortage in the funds required to provide existing members' benefits out of the contributions of new members, thus depriving the latter of any prospect of receiving the benefits for which they contribute. It is obvious that no person would join a society in such circumstances if the position were explained to him, and to induce him to do so in ignorance is obviously improper.

EXTRACT FOR THE YEAR 1929.

In cases where it has been found necessary to deal with a valuation deficiency by means of an increase of contributions or a reduction of benefits, the Registrar has sometimes found it necessary to suggest to a society the advisability of separate provision for future entrants. Many societies now find it difficult to secure new entrants even when the condition of the society is flourishing. It is obviously much more difficult to secure members if the new entrants are expected to shoulder part of a heavy deficiency by accepting a relatively low rate of benefit from the commencement of their membership. Nor is it always reasonable to assume that the conditions which have produced a deficiency in the past will operate in the future, e.g. bad investments or defalcations of officers. Consequently, where it is necessary to make adjustments in the rates of contribution or benefit, in order to meet a deficiency, it is usually desirable to make separate provision for new entrants. This is not infrequently overlooked by officers of societies and valuers.

In the case of a few small branches it was observed that the deficiency could only be met by very drastic reductions of benefits, if they were to maintain their separate existence. In these circumstances the Order Secretary was approached with the object of discovering whether something could not be done by way of amalgamation or transfer of engagements.

It is pleasing to be able to record that in an increasing number of cases the financial position seems to require attention not because it is bad, but because the accumulated surplus appears to be unnecessarily large. In such cases the Registrar has called attention to the advice of the valuer that benefits might be safely increased and in some of these cases the necessary amendments of rules have already been registered.

EXTRACT FOR THE YEAR 1935.

It is a matter of some satisfaction that, in spite of the tendency for sickness claims to increase in many societies, and the increase in net liability brought about as a result of providing for this factor, improved vitality, and falling interest rates, the financial position of societies as a whole has continued to improve. This is due largely to the fact that considerable profits continue to be derived (1) by reason of the actual sickness claims in many societies being less than the valuation provision made therefor (2) in societies providing death benefits only, from the great improvement in vitality in recent years and (3) by reason of the interest income of many societies being markedly greater than the valuation requirements. Further, in many cases where a deficiency has been revealed by valuation, a substantial reduction thereof has been effected by modification of the members' contracts. There is no doubt that most societies have a fuller appreciation of the significance of their periodical valuations than was formerly the case, the result being a greater readiness to take steps to deal with valuation deficiencies. This state of affairs is in some measure due to the action of the Registrar in directing the attention of societies to their valuation results and advising that steps be taken to liquidate deficiencies where such are disclosed. It is a source of satisfaction that in most cases the necessity for action is realised and modifications of the members' contracts are put into force. In some cases, however, the members refuse to take any steps towards restoring the solvency of their society although the deficiency disclosed is substantial. The result of this refusal to face the facts is that in due course the funds are liable to be absorbed by the comparatively heavy claims of the older members for sick and funeral benefits, so that the younger members, when they approach old age and require the benefits for which they have been contributing for many years, will find that the requisite funds are not available.

As an appendix to the chapter I give a summary, extracted from the Government's Actuary's reports, of the number and membership of Approved Societies as a whole.

(Statement B)

SUMMARY OF NUMBER OF SOCIETIES VALUED AS SEPARATE UNITS FOR NATIONAL HEALTH INSURANCE ADMINISTRATION, AND OF THE MEMBERSHIP AS AT THE DATE OF EACH VALUATION.

	NO. OF UNITS VALUED					NUMBER OF MEMBERS 000's					
						1st Valuation			2nd Valuation		
	1st Val.	2nd Val.	3rd Val.	4th Val.	5th Val.	Men	Women	Total	Men	Women	Total
Friendly Societies with branches ..	8,599	7,022	6,566	5,970	5,720	(not available)		3,472	2,391	758	3,149
Friendly Societies without branches	1,167	843	784	743	666			4,181	2,542	1,014	3,556
Industrial assurance and Collecting Societies	36	32	40	37	37			6,930	3,808	3,059	6,867
Trades Unions	252	160	149	138	129			1,531	1,271	242	1,513
Employers Provident Funds ..	108	78	69	67	55			137	81	32	113
Totals	10,162	8,135	7,608	6,955	6,607			16,251	10,093	5,105	15,198

	NUMBER OF MEMBERS 000's								
	3rd Valuation			4th Valuation			5th Valuation		
	Men	Women	Total	Men	Women	Total	Men	Women	Total
Friendly Societies with branches	2,358	790	3,148	2,238	736	2,974	2,232	774	3,006
Friendly Societies without branches ..	2,781	1,181	3,962	3,154	1,440	4,594	3,467	1,670	5,137
Industrial assurance and Collecting Societies	4,377	3,305	7,682	4,642	3,225	7,867	5,120	3,344	8,464
Trades Unions	1,221	254	1,475	1,173	260	1,433	1,184	289	1,473
Employers Provident Funds	81	32	113	53	32	85	54	34	88
Totals	10,818	5,562	16,380	11,260	5,693	16,953	12,057	6,111	18,168

Chapter V

Administration

(a) *The Societies*

(b) *The Department*

Introductory Note.

The question of the administration of the National Health Insurance scheme by the approved societies was one of the matters which received close attention in the Report of the Royal Commission, 1926, and I have had much in mind the views expressed in that report in preparing the material for this chapter.

The interim report of the Departmental Committee on Approved Society Finance and Administration 1916 (Cd. 8251) contains the main recommendations of that committee, but these deal for the most part with the financial provisions of the Acts and the general financial structure. Amongst the recommendations were those for the establishment of contingencies funds, special risks funds, and provisions for releasing part of the contributions carried to the sinking fund for the redemption of reserve values. The compulsory separation of men's and women's funds was not proposed, but it was recommended that facilities for separation should be afforded where desired by the society. As the recommendations of this important Committee, so far as they were adopted, have long since been merged in the general financial scheme of the Act, it is no longer of interest to examine the proposals in any detail.

In the second part of this chapter, the regulations governing the affairs of approved societies to which reference is made are consolidated in the N.H.I. Approved Societies Regulations, 1938 (S.R.O. 1938 No. 257).

(a) *Administration by the Societies.*

When the 1911 Bill became law, the machinery used for the administration of the scheme was that which was already in existence. Friendly Societies, Trade Unions, and Industrial Assurance Companies covered the whole country with their operations and it was the simplest plan, and probably the most economical in the circumstances, to make use of that machinery. When, in due course, provision for Widows and Orphans was added, the machinery which existed before 1911, that is, the Old Age (non-contributory) Pension machinery, was already centrally administered by the Government, and the administration of the Widows and Orphans pensions scheme and that of the contributory Old Age pensions were similarly centralised. It is a fair assumption that if we had been starting from nothing in 1911, the machine to be created to administer the National Health Insurance scheme would not have been anything like the organization which in fact administered it.

In the Report of the Royal Commission, it was suggested that the adoption of the Approved Society system was not merely imposed on Parliament in 1911 as an essential condition of a workable scheme in the conditions of the time, but that it was justified by the necessity of retaining under a scheme imposed by the State the general features of a system of insurance which had been evolved by the people themselves in their voluntary and unprompted efforts to meet their own requirements.

The Royal Commission received very little evidence of criticism with regard to the administration of sickness and disablement benefits and the conditions to be complied with by insured persons in order to obtain those benefits. The question of the extent to which the system of administration by approved societies might be open to criticism appears to have been examined on the following grounds:—

(1) The theory of government by the members,
(2) The size of the units engaged in the administration,
(3) The geographical distribution of the members, and
(4) The unfairness of a system which gives additional benefits varying widely in return for a flat contribution.

(1) *The theory of government by the members.*

The Act makes express provision that the constitution of every approved society "must provide for its affairs being subject to the absolute control of its members." This theory of self-government by the members owes its existence to the fact that it was originally contemplated that the National Health Insurance scheme could be administered by the old self-governing bodies—the Friendly Societies and the Trade Unions—and that they would be able to bring within the fold of their membership no less than two-thirds of the whole working population who had not hitherto practised the art of voluntary insurance or of self-government in any way. The Royal Commission in its report makes short work of the failure of this theory of self-government. It is really expecting too much of human nature to suppose that members compulsorily insured in a national scheme would take the slightest interest in the sickness benefit of their fellows, and the complete apathy of the insured population has from the outset been an acknowledged fact. The Royal Commission expresses no surprise whatever as to this, and says that it is not only contrary to human nature to expect anything else, but contrary to the whole experience of the interest that is taken by the community in affairs administered on a large scale, with the possible exception of a Parliamentary election. We have already noticed the lack of interest now almost universal even amongst the members of the lodges of the old Friendly Societies. The former spirit of membership and friendly interest displayed in the working of these local lodges has practically disappeared, and this is to some extent true of the smaller clubs and local societies. It was indeed quite visionary and impracticable to suppose that these small societies and local clubs could have ever roped into their membership the whole of the working population, and the theory of self-government was hardly worth retaining when this became apparent. But even where to a limited extent the small societies, and particularly the local societies, did enter upon the administration of the scheme, we have noticed elsewhere that the numbers of these societies has gradually declined, and that quite a considerable proportion of them have either completely disappeared or have merged their affairs in larger societies and so lost their identity.

It is really rather piquant that the Act should have provided for the affairs of every approved society being subject to the absolute control of its members and then perforce to have admitted to the administration the Industrial Assurance Companies and the Collecting Societies. And although the Royal Commission thought that there might be some advantage in having in the constitution of these large societies some provision for the control of the societies' affairs by the members if the occasion should arise, it requires a considerable amount of imagination to see how the control of a society with two or three million members could be effectively carried out if the occasion did arise. In the case of two of the largest of the Collecting Societies, it had been thought desirable to provide for control by the members by the establishment of a system of delegates elected at local meetings. This looks well on paper, but I had occasion to make an exhaustive investigation into the affairs of a large collecting society which had an annual and costly meeting of delegates who were supposed to have been appointed by the members. I found that, almost without exception—again owing to the apathy of the insured members—the delegates had been nominated years ago by the agents and re-appointed year after year as a matter of routine. The annual meeting of the delegates was almost a solemn farce and a sheer waste of the insured persons' money. In so far as these delegates exercised control over the committee of management, common-sense appeared to indicate that the committee might have been given an uninterrupted run for at least a quinquennial valuation period before the management by the executive of the affairs of the society came up for overhaul. I am therefore satisfied that the control of the affairs of a large society by the members does not cease to be less of a farce because "delegates" have annual meetings at delectable seaside resorts.

The Royal Commission, having made it clear beyond any possibility of doubt that self-government was a dead letter, proceeded to say that there was no great harm, and there might be some advantage, in the existence of the large societies provided they are efficiently and economically managed. With regard to the question of the constitution furnishing effective means for the control of the societies' affairs by the members if occasion should arise, there was clearly room for improvement, said the Royal Commission, and it was recommended that in connection with any general review of the rules of the societies, a society whose rules were found not to provide effective means by which the members could exercise control if they desired to do so should be required to amend its constitution in this respect. It is difficult to understand why the Royal Commission should have made this recommendation, or what was particularly in the mind of the members of the Commission with regard to deficiencies in the provisions for self-government. In the Act itself, after it had been decided to admit the large industrial companies and collecting societies, provision was made for the establishment by these large bodies of separate sections which became the approved societies, and it is within the recollection of those who were engaged in the establishment of the scheme that every device which it was possible to invent was resorted to in order to make it clear in the rules of these societies that they were under the government of the members.

(2) *The size of the units engaged in the administration.*

With regard to this question the attention of the Royal Commission was directed, by witnesses appearing on behalf of the central department, and others, to the extra work in accounting, auditing, and in general supervision necessitated by the existence of nearly 8,000 separate financial and valuation units. It would seem to be fairly obvious that the excessive number of small societies with their multiplication of establishment charges could not fail to be an expensive method of administration. There was, however, no evidence placed before the Commission that the larger societies were administered at a lower expense per head to their members than the small societies. Regulations fix the maximum amount per head that might be spent on expenses of administration, and the Commission found that, so far as savings within this limit provide a criterion of relative cost, the general body of small societies and branches did not show to any disadvantage.

(3) *The geographical distribution of members of Approved Societies.*

Closely allied to the criticism that the approved society system is unduly costly in administration—indeed one of the causes for this alleged expensiveness—is the overlapping of effort arising from the fact that approved societies may carry on business in any part of the country. In any moderate-sized town the insured persons may be scattered amongst some hundreds of societies and branches, each of which has to make arrangements for the administration of the cash benefits to members entitled to them. Statements were made in evidence before the Royal Commission that there were 488 societies with members in Liverpool, that in Bolton there were 285 societies operating, in Brighton 304, Norwich 213, and so on. As an example of a large number of societies possessing a ludicrously small membership in a particular district, Dundee was quoted, where there were 217 separate societies (ignoring branches), of which 99 had less than 10 members in the town, and 52 had one member only. These societies had their head offices at London, Manchester, Glasgow, Aberdeen, Edinburgh, Leeds, Portsmouth, Newcastle, Tunbridge Wells, etc. The process of the gradual disappearance of the small society goes on, but only affects this question of overlapping to a limited extent.

The Royal Commission recognised that this criticism went to the root of the question whether the present organisation should be continued, at the same time expressing the view that its importance might be easily over-estimated. The chief criterion must be the effect upon the insured person. On this the Commission received no evidence that the insured person who migrated from one district to another suffered delay in the receipt of benefit, or other inconvenience, from the fact that the office, or head office, as the case may be, of his society was not in the area in which he resided. It may indeed be, said the Royal Commission, that in this respect the existence of large centralised societies with offices and representatives in every industrial centre in the country, is a positive advantage, since the member of such a society is sure of the means by which his needs may be attended to wherever he may be; in any case, the insured person who suffered inconvenience had the remedy in his own hands, since he could transfer to a society of his choice.

The manifest absurdity of a system which permits of the existence of a large number of societies in one town, each society having in that place one or two members only, must give to the student of administration something of a shock, and he is tempted to reflect that the Royal Commission dismissed this ground of criticism rather light-heartedly. If it is agreed, as it must be, that it is a matter of indifference to the vast majority of insured persons what particular society they belong to, it must also be agreed that where you have a national scheme in which everyone is compulsorily insured, the scheme must be administered with due regard to the convenience of the insured person, and also with due regard to the importance of economical administration. An insured person would probably be prepared to go to a local office to collect his sickness benefit, in precisely the same way that he would go to the post office for his pension or to buy a postal order. It is fair to recognise that he would prefer to have his sickness benefit brought round to him and his contribution card collected by the agent of a centralised society, as this would involve him in no inconvenience whatsoever, and it is not to be supposed that under a centrally administered scheme directed by the government, or by the local authority, the insured person would be likely to enjoy the advantages of having his sick pay brought to him, and his cards collected in this way. From the point of view of economical administration it is obvious that if fifty societies are operating in a town each with one or two members, they cannot mantain local offices, and equally they can have no system in that town of supervision by sick visitors—which is recognised as an essential feature of the administration of sickness benefit.

The geographical distribution of members under the present system can only stand condemned, and the maintenance of the system must be justified on other grounds, such as, if we are to be frank, the ground of political expediency.

(4) *The unfairness of a system which gives additional benefits varying widely in return for a flat contribution.*

This, the principal ground on which the Approved Society

system was criticised, was examined in the Royal Commission's report at some length.

It was contended that the inequalities in the benefits to which members of different societies are entitled are too great to be defensible in a State scheme of insurance based on compulsory contributions at a uniform rate. This result was claimed, however, by others as an advantage of the system, in that it enables the insured to group themselves in such a way as to secure the maximum advantage from their contributions and so to neutralise whatever inequality would result from the application of a flat-rate contribution to all insured persons, regardless of the variations in their several risks as affected by occupation or environment, or in their economic condition either as classes or individuals.

Where the members of a society followed the same trade or calling in which there was a heavy incidence of sickness, they could not understand why, in a national scheme, the burden should not be nationally distributed. The Scottish Miners' Federation said that " no one marvels at the volume of pardonable misunderstanding and personal resentment of the insured person regarding the provision of additional benefits. He never can grasp the justice of an arrangement that gives 15/- worth of sickness benefit a week in one society and 20/- a week in some other society for the flat contribution of 10d. a week. He regards the question as incapable of intelligent explanation and despairingly concludes that these disparities are nothing more or less than the product of an invisible evil genius."

The conclusion of the Royal Commission (p.118) was that with a flat rate of contribution from all insured persons, whatever their liability to sickness, the provision of varying benefits can be justified. They were impressed by the fact that the inequality of experience between different societies was accompanied by a considerable inequality in wages. For example, agricultural workers who received lower wages than the average artisans show better results under National Health Insurance. It was mainly on the ground that agricultural workers are on the whole less liable to sickness than persons engaged in other occupations that a demand was made on their behalf in 1911 for a lower rate of contribution and it was chiefly on the ground of the administrative difficulties of differentiation in the rate of contribution that this demand was resisted.

Another justification of differentiation in benefits lies in the incentive which is thereby offered to good and careful administration. It would be bad both administratively and financially if the persons charged with the responsibility for considering claims for benefit felt that there was nothing to be gained by doing their work well and thoroughly.

At the same time, the Commission inclined to the view that (p.115) "even if it were possible hypothetically to assume a uniform standard of administration throughout all societies, the discrepancies which would have resulted would have been almost as great as those which have in fact emerged (on valuation), and we are strengthened in this view by the consideration that there are prosperous societies in which administration is not strict and unfortunate societies which are unfortunate despite strictness of supervision."

The approved society system of administering a national scheme can only be justified on grounds of expediency, but with such a system—the societies competing in the field for new members—it can only be said that varying scales of benefits, whatever the merits of the case, are inevitable.

A further ground on which the approved society system was criticised was that it "stands in the way of the unification of social insurance which so many people now desire". In support of this, appeal was made to the fact that the societies had not been considered to be suitable bodies for the administration of Unemployment Insurance or of the newly-introduced scheme for Widows, Orphans and Old Age Pensions. It was suggested that "the present approved society system is not suitable for administering any other form of insurance benefit, nor does it seem capable of being co-ordinated with any other system of administration". The Royal Commission with regard to this says (p.99):

"We cannot say that criticisms of this kind commend themselves to our judgment. We have not been asked to consider the unification of social insurance, and while we cannot regard it as a practicable or desirable development merely because so many people are said to desire it, we equally cannot assume, in the absence of evidence directed to the point, that if it were introduced, no place in its administration could be found for the approved societies. If there are grounds for concluding that the approved societies system is well adapted to administer the benefits of National Health Insurance, it does not appear to us that the societies should be dispossessed from this work because some other forms of organisation are better fitted to administer other branches of social activity. The assumption implied in these criticisms that one form of organisation could equally well administer these diverse schemes of social welfare, appears to us to take for granted much that should be investigated before an opinion is formed." In conclusion, the Royal Commission states (p.102):

"We have to take note of the fact that the Approved Societies are in possession of the field, by the action of Parliament, that they have their organisations widely distributed over the whole of the country and their staffs trained in the details of what, in many respects, is an intricate piece of social administration. The onus of showing that the system, either from causes inherent in itself, or from personal shortcomings of those by whom it is operated, works so imperfectly that it ought to be abolished, rests upon those who take this view. We have considered their evidence with care, and we trust, without bias. In the result we have come to the conclusion that no case for the abolition of the societies can be established on the broad ground of defects and shortcomings in administration. In saying this we are not to be understood as indicating that there are no faults to be remedied. We could wish, for instance, that in some quarters the interests of the insured persons were more fully considered in regard to such matters as expenditure on administration within the prescribed limit, or that the rights of the members had been more fully respected when the constitutions of certain of the societies were framed; and we have had occasional evidence, which must be treated with respect, pointing to shortcomings in the payment of benefits and other dealings between the societies and their members. But we realise that defects of these kinds spring less from improper motives than from those human weaknesses that in some form or other must reveal themselves in whatever type of organisation may be erected to administer a great scheme such as the one we have under review; and we cannot accept them as amounting, in the whole, to the establishment of such a case against the societies as to warrant us in recommending that they should be superseded."

"We do not" says the Royal Commission (p. 102) "think that the best interests either of the State or of the insured population would be served by a vast amalgamation of all of the resources of the Scheme in a common fund administered from the centre, and for the reason given we are satisfied that such an amalgamation would create as much discontent as it would allay. From this point of view, therefore, we have come to the conclusion that a system of self-governing bodies is to be preferred and should be retained."

And finally (p. 103)—

"It must be clearly understood that our recommendation is made in relation to the scheme of National Health Insurance as it exists at present, and that our view in favour of the retention of Approved Societies does not necessarily imply that developments in the system of social insurance outside the range of present contemplation might not necessitate a reconsideration of the position."

(*b*) *The control of the Department.*

Just as in the case of the direction of the affairs of the society the pleasant fiction is preserved that those affairs are subject to the absolute control of its insured members, so with regard to the control exercised by the Ministry of Health and the Department of Health for Scotland the theory is preserved that each society is left with a considerable measure of autonomy. This was in substance stated in the official evidence put before the Royal Commission on National Health Insurance. It is doubtless true that the constitution of societies and the machinery by which they carry out their functions vary widely. The Department is not concerned to interfere with such questions as appointment of staff, or the particular channel through which the benefits are distributed. But it would be conceded, after examining the provisions of the Approved Societies Regulations, 1938, with their 236 clauses and numerous schedules, that the control by the Departments is in all essentials complete. And indeed this is inevitable in a national scheme financed by compulsory contributions from a very large proportion of the adult population, employers and employed, and with Exchequer assistance. The standard benefits are fixed and uniform. The additional benefits which may be provided out of surpluses can only be administered under schemes which require the approval of the Department. The amount which may be expended on administration is limited by regulation. Amongst some of the provisions contained in the regulations, we may note the following:

(Art. 13) Upon application from the society, the Minister

issues such moneys "as are shown to his satisfaction to be necessary to meet expenditure properly incurred."

(Art. 22) The Minister transfers to the investments account under his complete control one half of the sums available for investment in the case of each society, and he may also invest the whole of the sums if the society so requests.

(Art. 29) The whole of the contribution cards of the members of the society are forwarded to the Department at the end of each half yearly period, and the society must furnish such summaries, declarations and returns as the Department may require.

(Art. 41) The society must keep such books and accounts as the Minister may direct.

(Third schedule, paragraph 2c) The amount which may be expended on administration must not exceed 4s./6d. per head of membership per annum.

(Art. 57) If a joint management account is kept in which the affairs of the voluntary and state business are merged, or a contract administration payment is made to the parent body, the request for this course must be supported by resolutions of a special meeting of which notice has been given.

(Art. 162) The society must not establish branches without the Minister's consent.

(Art. 173) Any party to a dispute under the rules of the society may appeal to the Minister.

There are also elaborate provisions dealing with amalgamation and transfer of engagements, with mal-administration, with withdrawal of approval, with the cessation, expulsion, and the dissolution of branches. If the society is found to be mal-administering its affairs, the Minister may appoint a manager.

It is hardly necessary to labour the point that the control of the Department is complete, and that this is inevitable. Nor can there be any question that a sense of responsibility in the administration of a vast national scheme has developed and matured amongst the several types of societies engaged in the administration of the scheme, and that the control of the Department, which has always been exercised with the advice and assistance of a strong advisory committee representative of the different types of society, has had valuable reactions on the administration of the societies in the wider fields in which the Department has no concern.

CHAPTER VI.

FINANCE.

(*a*) *Cost of Administration.*

(*b*) *Benefits—Estimates and Experience.*

(*a*) Cost of Administration.

It had been my purpose to examine the question of the cost of administration, first, by looking at the expenditure of the societies, and then at the cost of that part of the activities of the central departments which is properly appropriated to the administration of National Health Insurance. I have, however, come to the conclusion that this separation of the expenditure would not serve any useful purpose, and that the cost of the administration as a whole has to be looked at. This is set out in the following statement which has been extracted from the Report of Expenditure on Public Social Services, issued in November 1937, (Cmd. 5609). It will be seen that the cost of administration is 14.9 per cent. of the total expenditure on benefits, and that this is very high as compared with the percentage in the case of the schemes which are centrally administered,—9.7 and 9.2 in the case of the Uemployment Benefit and Unemployment Assistance schemes, respectively, and the very small figures of 2.9, 2.5 and 1.5 in the case of the pensions schemes.

Pensions administration affords no criterion by reference to which the matter can be examined. The fact of death or the attainment of a certain age involves one claim on each policy or contract, which, of course, has to be exhaustively examined at the time. But afterwards there is the merest routine machinery for paying out benefit until the end; whereas, in the case of sickness and disablement benefits claims are made continuously in a large proportion of cases and constantly recur in the case of the same individual throughout the whole period of insurance, and this involves a vast checking machinery. It would on the other hand probably be found, as the result of an intensive research into the question, that the cost of administration of National Health Insurance might very fairly be compared with the cost of the administration of the Unemployment schemes which are administered by the central departments with their staffs spread all over

EXTRACT FROM RETURN OF EXPENDITURE ON PUBLIC SOCIAL SERVICES FOR THE FINANCIAL YEAR 1935 (NOVEMBER, 1937). CMD. 5609.

ENGLAND AND WALES AND SCOTLAND.

		£000's Administration expenses	Percentage of total	Benefits, etc.	£000's Total
(*a*) Unemployment Insurance, etc., Acts.					
(i) Unemployment Benefit, etc.	E	4,092		37,834	41,926
	S	517		5,101	5,618
		5,609	9·7	42,935	47,544*
(ii) Unemployment Allowances and Transitional Payments	E	3,559		35,339	38,898
	S	729		7,228	7,957
		4,288	9·2	42,567	46,855
(*b*) National Health Insurance Acts	E	5,097		29,116	34,213
	S	602		3,529	4,131
		5,699	14·9	32,645	38,344
(*c*) Widows', Orphans' and Old Age Contributory Pensions Acts	E	1,137		38,670	39,807
	S	141		4,680	4,821
		1,278	2·9	43,350	44,628
(*d*) Old Age Pensions Acts	E	602		38,488	39,090
	S	72		4,612	4,684
		674	1·5	43,100	43,774
(*e*) War Pensions Acts and the Ministry of Pensions Act	E	900		35,491	36,391
	S	107		3,952	4,059
		1,007	2·5	39,443	40,450
Totals for these services . .		17,555	6·7	244,040	261,595

*There was also loan expenditure (interest and repayments) not included here.

E England and Wales. S Scotland.

the country. Admittedly the subjects of sickness and unemployment involve wholly different checks and investigations, but from close personal contact with both subjects, I should venture the opinion that the investigation of claims for unemployment benefit and unemployment assistance involves at least as much labour and detail as the investigation of claims for sickness benefits.

Within the total cost of the administration of the Health Insurance scheme it is worthy of note that the cost of local administration in the case of medical benefit, where there is a geographical distribution of the administering bodies—the Insurance

Committees—according to county and county borough areas, is as follows. (The figures for England, from the 18th annual report of the Minister of Health 1936/7 (Cmd 5516) Appx. XXXII are sufficient for the purpose).

Medical benefit £9,234,000—cost of administration by Insurance Committees £370,000, approximately 4 per cent.

Cash benefits for the same period £18,220,000—cost of administration by the Approved Societies £3,520,000, or nearly 20 per cent.

It must be fairly recognised that the Approved Societies have considerable expenditure in furnishing records to the Insurance Committees for the purposes of medical benefit which strictly ought to be shown as part of the administrative expenditure on medical benefit; and admittedly the relative duties involved in administering cash benefits and medical benefit are of a different character and extent. But it is really difficult to suppose that if the medical benefit can be administered at a cost of 4 per cent., the 20 per cent. charge for administration of the cash benefits is justified.

The observation made above as to the relative cost involved in examining claims for pensions as compared with the cost of dealing with claims for sickness benefit throughout the whole period of insurance may fairly apply to the cost of administering death benefits or life insurance or endowment policies. If, on the one hand, we find such a heavy expenditure on the cash benefits administered by Approved Societies as compared with unemployment benefits administered by a central department, it is even more disturbing to turn from the cost of administration of Health Insurance to the cost of Industrial Assurance, notwithstanding the substantial economies effected.

Reference may be made to the statement given in Appendix No. 2 for information as to the ratio of expenses to premiums between the years 1917 and 1936. It will be seen that the actual proportion of expenses to premiums was 40.77 in 1917, and had fallen to 33.75 in 1936.

The industrial insurance premium income of the group of offices associated with the National Amalgamated Approved Society has grown in twenty-five years more than threefold, and the funds nearly tenfold, and in the same period it would appear that there has been a total reduction in the rate of expenses equal to 13 per cent. of the premium income.

In the case of the Prudential Societies the cost of administration has come down from 44 per cent. to 22 per cent. in the last twenty-five years. This reduction, it is understood, was largely due to reorganisation, particularly putting the agents on a whole time basis. The Royal Commission report makes a full reference to the question of the system under which a lump sum payment for administration is made by the Approved Societies to the parent bodies. It has been noted earlier in this paper that the large industrial offices set up separate sections, with provisions for self-government, in order to comply with the requirements of the Act. The Approved Society, in these cases, usually makes a lump sum payment for administration to the parent body equivalent to the maximum sum which is allowed (4s. 6d. a head) to Approved Societies under the regulations in respect of the cost of administration.

As the societies in which this arrangement obtains, although few in number, have an aggregate membership of nearly half the total insured population, the question as to the reasonableness of the arrangement for paying over the whole amount available in one sum is, it will be seen, a matter of some importance. Sir Walter Kinnear, in the course of his evidence before the Royal Commission, said on this subject:—

> "We have simply to look at the cost of that Society (the Prudential) as compared with the cost of other Societies, and endeavour as best we can to decide whether that lump sum which is agreed upon is a fair and equitable amount. I do not think the system has been abused; I do not think that the Society is placed at any serious disadvantage by the arrangements; but, of course, it is open to the criticism that there is a very considerable expenditure over which we have no supervision or no auditorial rights."

The Royal Commission report, looking at the case of the Prudential Approved Societies, says, "that sums totalling nearly £700,000 a year are paid out of the State Insurance funds to the Prudential Insurance Company, and these payments appear as single items in the accounts of the Approved Societies as submitted to the Treasury Auditor and to the insured members, no details being available of the manner in which the money is applied by the company. We feel, therefore, that a serious responsibility rests upon the Central Departments to scrutinise closely the terms and conditions of any proposed arrangement of this kind before giving their approval.

"We questioned witnesses representing the Prudential Approved Societies on the subject, and it appeared from their evidence that, although a considerable reduction has recently been effected in the overhead charges of the parent company as a result of certain measures of reorganisation, that reduction had not been reflected in the amount paid by the company by the Approved Societies. We feel that it is only reasonable that the insured members of the Societies should receive some compensating advantage under arrangements of this character in return for their surrender of their ordinary right of scrutinising and criticising the detailed expenditure of the Society's funds for purposes of administration, and we think that before giving their approval to such arrangements, the Central Department should take all possible steps to satisfy themselves that this will be secured."

It may be open to doubt whether, since the date of the report of the Royal Commission, any reduction has in fact been made in the amount paid to the parent company by the Approved Societies. The parent company could reasonably urge that even though the cost of administration of the affairs of the Prudential Societies as a whole had been very materially reduced it was still in excess of the amount allowed to Approved Societies generally for the expenses of administration and that, therefore, there was no unfairness to the members of the Approved Societies in having to pay over for administration a proportion of the premium income which represented less than the actual cost to the parent body.

The Royal Commission made reference to the fact that the question of the sums to be made available to Approved Societies for administration was the subject of close enquiry by a Departmental Committee in 1921, and the Commission was satisfied that the evidence heard on the subject was not such as to warrant any reconsideration of the matter.

No attempt appears to have been made by the Commission to investigate the question whether the cost of administration might be materially reduced under an entirely different system, but as the view had elsewhere been expressed in the report that the system of administration by the Approved Societies could not be disturbed the question of the cost under another system might well be regarded as one merely of academic interest. The Report finds that in general the rate of allowance for administration was sufficient, and no evidence appears to have been tendered to the Commission by the Departments or otherwise that the rate was excessive.

(b) Benefits—Estimates and Experience.

Before examining the main question which is the subject of this section, I have thought that it would be of interest to show how weekly contributions in the National Health Insurance scheme are disposed of. It is a simple question to which, I fear, it is only possible to give a complex answer, but I have endeavoured to reduce the answer to the simplest possible proportions. I have relied for my calculations on statistics which relate to England and Wales only; it would not make any material difference to the results if the figures for Scotland had also been examined.

I have decided that, rather than split up the contribution with meticulous calculations involving decimals, it would be better to express the income from contributions as £1,000 and show the other figures of receipts and expenditure in relation to this amount of £1,000. On this basis, and taking the average of the five years 1931—1935, the receipts and payments have been as follows:—

(The contributions are the combined payments by employers and employed; the exchequer does not pay any proportion of the contributions but pays a proportion of the cost of benefits as they materialise),

RECEIPTS:	£
Contributions	1,000
Exchequer	243
..	1,243
Interest on accumulated funds ..	227
Total receipts	£1,470
PAYMENTS:	
Cash benefits:	£
Sickness	404
Disablement	235
Maternity	64
Other benefits ..	103
	806
Medical benefit	390
	1,196
Administration	212
Total expenditure on benefits and administration	£1,408
Excess of receipts over expenditure (or a little over 4%)	£62

It will be observed from this table that the income derived from the contributions from the insured persons and their employers together with the proportion of benefits paid by the exchequer—£1,243—are jointly insufficient to meet the cost of benefits and of administration—£1,408—The interest on the accumulated funds of the approved societies—£227—is required in part for benefits and administration, and a balance of £62 remains to carry to the accumulated funds.

The actual increase in the accumulated funds during the five years referred to has been approximately £5,000,000; this is derived entirely from the part of the interest on previous accumulated funds in the possession of the approved societies in so far as this interest has not been used up in the payment of benefits and the cost of administration.

For the purposes of this section of the chapter, I have made reference to the reports of the Actuaries in relation to the scheme of insurance embodied in the National Insurance Bill, 1911 (Cd 5681), and a further report of the Actuaries in relation to the Bill as amended in Committee (Cd 5983), and also to the several reports of the Government Actuary on the valuations of Approved Societies. The estimates given by the Actuaries in their original calculations as to the number of compulsory contributors becoming members of Approved Societies is set out in the following statement, which is not carried beyond the year 1927/8:—

Year	Men	Women	Both Sexes
1912-13 ..	8,579,000	3,628,000	12,207,000
1917-18 ..	9,586,000	4,020,000	13,606,000
1922-23 ..	10,412,000	4,355,000	14,767,000
1927-28 ..	11,211,000	4,687,000	15,898,000

Notwithstanding the disturbing effects of the War 1914-18 and the subsequent industrial situation, it is of interest to compare these estimates of the insured population with the following statement showing the numbers and distribution of the insured population as at the fourth valuation of Approved Societies. The number of men in the original estimate for 1927/8 corresponds with remarkable closeness to the actual number of men in insurance at the time of valuation. In the case of the women, the number compulsorily insured is in excess of the original estimate by about 1,000,000. The figures given in the fourth valuation report of course include voluntary contributors, but these are not sufficiently large in relation to the whole to alter the value of the comparison.

NATIONAL DISTRIBUTION OF INSURED POPULATION AS AT THE FOURTH VALUATION.

Country	Men	Women	Total
England ..	9,234,075	4,770,868	14,004,943
Scotland ..	1,143,686	587,829	1,731,515
Wales ..	674,449	194,148	868,597
N. Ireland ..	207,885	140,206	348,091
Total ..	11,260,095	5,693,051	16,953,146

The figures for the Fifth Valuation may be noted—They are as follows:

Totals at Fifth Valuation	12,057,040	6,111,078	18,168,118

I have chosen the year 1927/8 for the purposes of comparison with the estimates because that was the last year for which the Actuaries in their original report ventured to make a forecast. The figures are as follows:—

EXPENDITURE ON BENEFITS, 1927-8.

£ MILLIONS

Benefits	England	Scotland	Total	Estimated cost
Sickness ..	10·2	1·1	11·3	10·2
Disablement ..	5·5	·7	6·2	4·5
Maternity ..	1·5	·2	1·7	—
Medical ..	9·1	1·0	10·1	—
Administration	4·7	·5	5·2	—

The estimated cost of sickness and disablement benefit was set out in the Actuaries' report on the National Insurance Bill, 1911, as presented to the House of Commons (Cd 5681).

The amounts set out in that report have been loaded by 50 per cent. for the purposes of comparison with the actual expenditure because the rates of benefit were increased since the War (1914-18) by approximately that amount.

The expenditure on maternity benefit does not call for any comment here. The figures have been fairly steady through the whole period of years.

The original estimate of the cost of medical benefit was based on a figure of 6/- a head, including drugs. This became out of date before medical benefit came into operation, and the cost has varied from time to time with the population and the capitation rate negotiated with the doctors.

Similarly, the cost of administration would vary with the population and the amounts per head agreed to be allowed to the approved societies.

The cost of the sickness and disablement benefits varies of necessity over a considerable period owing to causes other than those which have a direct relationship to the number of the insured population. The cost of the other benefits, maternity and medical, varies directly with the insured population and, in the case of medical benefit, also with the capitation rate negotiated from time to time with the medical profession. The question of the control of sickness and disablement benefits is dealt with in the next chapter; it is of interest here, looking at the matter broadly, to examine the valuation reports of the Government Actuary and see what has emerged at the several valuations. I have, therefore, prepared some extensive extracts from these reports which must speak for themselves. The vast surpluses disclosed on valuation, and the amounts which the Actuary has been able to certify as disposable, although very largely affected by other factors and especially by the rate of interest obtainable on investment during the valuation periods, undoubtedly suggest that the expenditure on sickness and disablement benefits has not greatly outrun the estimates. How far this justifies the assumption that sickness claims have, on the whole, been well controlled, is a question meriting more intensive inquiry. There is no doubt that more investigation and research into insurance sickness, as suggested in Sir I. G. Gibbon's paper on the public social services, is desirable. "There have," he says, "been disquieting increases, and though much of this may be because the insured have become more "treatment-conscious," to use modern slang, some of it is due to malingering, probably substantial in the aggregate but not proportionately, and possibly still more to valetudinarianism, far more insidious and dangerous than deliberate malingering because unconsciously weakening the will to resistance of disease.

The present administration of health insurance, admirable as it is from the static standpoint, needs to be more dynamic."

The following statement illustrates the growth of the funds of the approved societies at the valuation dates and, owing especially to the importance of reserve values, it is essential that the valuation figures should be studied in the light of the notes which I have extracted from the several valuation reports. The summary of the statement of funds of the approved societies is followed immediately by a note on the process of valuation and by a summary of the valuation balance sheets as at the fifth valuation.

FUNDS OF APPROVED SOCIETIES AT THE VALUATION DATES.

	Reserve* Values. £	Investments and other Assets £	Reference to Report
1st Valuation	64,018,000	55,461,000	Cmd. 1662 (1922)
2nd Valuation	97,400,000	92,260,000	Cmd. 2785 (1927)
3rd Valuation	49,636,000	117,509,000	Cmd. 3978 (1931)
4th Valuation	47,774,000	116,589,000	Cmd. 5496 (1937)
5th Valuation	45,000,000	128,000,000	Cmd. 6455 (1943)

* Reserve Values are the capital sums required in respect of members entering insurance at ages over 16 to meet the estimated loss arising from the acceptance of such members by approved societies at the flat rate of contribution.

NOTES:

From 1st Valuation Report.

The position as to reserve values is as follows. The aggregate reserve values credited in respect of persons who became members of approved societies during the first fifteen months of the Act amounted to £69,500,000, and to these were added similar credits for subsequent entrants amounting to £16,000,000 making £85,500,000 in all. This sum was reduced by £15,900,000 in respect of the transfer values of persons who passed out of insurance otherwise than by death during the period, the net amount of reserve values credited being thus £69,600,000.

Under the provisions of the Acts, the Commissioners retain part of the contributions paid by insured persons and their employers for the provision of interest on, and for the redemption of, their liabilities in respect of reserve values. During the period up to December 1918, approved societies received from this source about £14,200,000 as interest and the sum of £5,600,000 was applied towards redemption. The aggregate amount of reserve values outstanding at the date of the valuation was accordingly reduced to £64,000,000.

From 2nd Valuation Report.

At 31st December 1918, the total funds of approved societies, including the funds relative to insured persons resident in the Irish Free State, amounted to about £119,500,000 of which £64 millions were represented by outstanding reserve values and the balance by investments and cash. The figure for outstanding reserve values was reduced by about £1 million in respect of alterations in membership prior to 1919, to which effect had not been given at the time of the first valuation. During the inter-valuation period approximately £50½ millions were credited to societies in respect of additional reserve values by the Acts of 1920 and 1922 ; and further credits of £13½ millions were made in respect of new entrants into insurance during the intervaluation period, thus making a total of £127 millions. This total was reduced by about £21 millions in respect of reserve values of persons who passed out of insurance otherwise than by death, while about £2½ millions were withdrawn in respect of societies in the Irish Free State, and £6 millions were converted into money by the redemption operations. The aggregate amount of reserve values outstanding at the second valuation was thus £97,400,000.

From 3rd Valuation Report.

At the second valuation the total funds of approved societies amounted to £189,660,000, of which £97,400,000 were represented by reserve values. These now stand at £49,636,000, the change being attritutable chiefly to cancelments, amounting to £39,300,000, to which effect was given as at 31st December 1925, following the net reduction of the liabilities of the approved societies by the termination at the age of 65 (instead of 70) of sickness and disablement benefits, and of contributions, under Section 37 of the Widows Orphans and Old Age Contributory Pensions Act 1925. The increase of monetary assets during the inter-valuation period was about £25¼ millions, the investments and cash in hand, etc., having grown from about £92¼ millions to £117½ millions.

From 4th Valuation Report.

The reduction of reserve values represents the net effect of redemptions of reserve values and of creations of new reserve values. An abnormal increase in the latter item for the year 1930, as a result of the admission of voluntary contributors under the terms of the Act of 1929 operated to delay the due redemption of outstanding reserve values.

It is perhaps desirable to point out that increase or otherwise in funds over a series of years does not, in itself, provide an indication of the strength of an insurance institution ; it is the function of the valuation to supply this. The small decline in the total funds of approved societies in the inter-valuation period is not, therefore, to be interpreted as a sign of deterioration in their financial position, e.g., the growth of societies' funds has been substantially and properly retarded as a result of the expenditure on additional benefits of at least £20,000,000 by societies during the inter-valuation period.

NOTE ON THE PROCESS OF VALUATION

Valuation, as applied to insurance institutions, is a measurement of future benefit payments on the one hand and of future contribution receipts on the other. It involves, in the first place, an estimate of the number of members of each present age who will survive to each future year until, within the lapse of time, the last survivor is dead, or has passed out of insurance from any other cause required to be recognised in the calculations. In the second place, when the number of persons surviving in insurance to each succeeding year has been estimated, it is necessary to calculate the amount of the claims these persons will make in the year and the amount of the contributions they will pay. In calculating the benefits to be drawn under the system of National Health Insurance, note must be taken of the ages to which the insured will have attained, for, except in the case of medical benefit, age is an important factor in this connection. Resort must be had, for example to tables of " sickness rates " to measure the charge for sickness and disablement benefits.

The actuary then obtains the " present value " of all the sums that will be paid in benefits and the " present value " of all the sums that will be received in contributions. Having obtained these values he is now in a position to prepare his valuation balance sheet, and this he does, so far as the system of National Health Insurance is concerned, by inserting on the one side the present value of the benefits to be drawn (including cost of administration) constituting the liabilities, and on the other side (i) the present value of the contributions to be paid in future, (ii) the present value of the State grants taken as a proportion of the benefits and (iii) the amount of the benefit fund on the valuation date. The sum of these three latter items constitute the assets. If these are greater than the liabilities there is a surplus ; if, on the other hand, the liabilities are the greater, there is a deficiency.

The summary of Valuation Balance Sheets at the Fifth Valuation is as follows :

FIFTH VALUATION.
SUMMARY OF VALUATION BALANCE SHEETS.

Liabilities		£ millions	Assets	£ millions
Present Value of Benefits and cost of Administration		596·9	Present Value of Contributions ..	366·9
	£		Present Value of State Grants ..	95·3
Surpluses	34·3		Total Benefit Funds	165·8
less deficiencies	·9		Grants under Section 150 of the National Health Insurance Act, 1936	1·1
Net Surplus		33·4	Other Assets	1·2
		£630·3		£630·3

I have extracted also from the valuation reports a statement of the valuation results showing surplus and deficiency and the amount of disposable surplus as at each valuation and, finally, a summary of the valuation results at the fourth valuation according to the type of society.

STATEMENT OF VALUATION RESULTS.

	Valuations shewing surplus. Total amount of surplus.			Valuations shewing deficiency. Total amount of deficiency		
	Men only £000's	Women only £000's	Men and women in common insurance £000's	Men only £000's	Women only £000's	Wen and women in common insurance. £000's
First Valuation	6,648	2,581	8,045	49	4	28
Second Valuation	16,289	5,181	20,944	42	16	34
Third Valuation	19,301	4,271	13,066	453	150	245
Fourth Valuation	20,716	6,374	10,395	298	342	101

Figures not given in the Actuary's abridged report on the Fifth Valuation.

DISPOSABLE SURPLUS

By Section 104 (2) of the N.H.I. Act, 1936, is is provided that where a surplus is found on valuation the valuer shall certify as disposable only such part of it as in his opinion, having regard to the circumstances and prospects of the society or branch, may reasonably be expended within the period of the duration of the scheme of additional benefits following the valuation.

	Amount of Net Surplus disclosed on valuation	Amount certified as "disposable"
	£	£
1st Valuation ..	17,274,000	9,184,000
2nd " ..	42,413,000	26,619,000
3rd " ..	35,791,000	19,811,000
4th " ..	36,743,000	20,105,000
5th " ..	33,094,000	18,823,000

SUMMARY OF VALUATION RESULTS ACCORDING TO TYPE OF SOCIETY

Fourth Valuation.*

	No. of Valuations shewing surplus			Amount of surplus.		
Group.	Men only	Women only	Men and women insured in the same society	Men only £000's	Women only £000's	Men and women insured in the same society £000's
Friendly Socs. with branches	2,287	484	2,753	3,341	575	5,497
Friendly Socs. without branches	222	74	393	5,988	1,747	3,490
Industrial Assurance and Collecting Socs. ..	10	8	8	8,601	3,919	40
Trade Unions	81	9	39	2,549	127	1,196
Employers' Provident Funds	22	2	43	236	7	172

SUMMARY OF VALUATION RESULTS ACCORDING TO TYPE OF SOCIETY

Fourth Valuation.

	No. of Valuations shewing deficiency			Amount of deficiency		
Group	Men only	Women only	Men & women insured in the same society	Men only £000's	Women only £000's	Men & women insured in the same society £000's
Friendly Socs. with branches	60	90	98	15	30	41
Friendly Socs. without branches	8	10	13	204	86	60
Industrial Assurance and Collecting Socs. ..	—	5	—	—	116	—
Trade Unions	4	3	1	80	110	1
Employers' Provident Funds	—	—	—	—	—	—

Note.—In addition 218 Valuations shewed equality of assets and liabilities.

* A similar analysis is not given in the abridged report on the Fifth Valuation.

To conclude this chapter on Finance I may perhaps refer to a memorandum, set out in appendix No. 4, with regard to the financial questions examined in the Report of the Royal Commission on National Health Insurance. This memorandum was prepared by me, shortly after the publication of the Report, for the information of the medical profession. It is only necessary to say that the recommendations of the Royal Commission, owing to the financial exigencies of the time and also, it cannot be questioned, to the opposition of approved societies to pooling one-half of their future surpluses, came to nought.

Chapter VII

The Control of Sickness Benefit Claims

So soon after the coming into operation of the National Insurance Act as August 1913 it was thought desirable to set up a departmental committee to enquire into the alleged excessive claims upon Approved Societies in respect of sickness benefit. That committee reported in July 1914 but, as immediately afterwards the War broke out, it was not possible to give effect to its findings and recommendations for some years. The committee in general terms reported that, notwithstanding the difficulties involved in bringing the Act into operation, the machinery of administration had been working as smoothly as could reasonably have been anticipated, that officials of Approved Societies had shown zeal in promoting the prosperous working of the Act, and that in general the medical profession had brought to their work a desire to do their best for their patients. The committee also found that there was little if any evidence of fraud on the part of insured persons, or of deliberate malingering, but considerable evidence of a tendency to take the utmost advantage of the benefits under the Act, to claim for trivial complaints, and to prolong unduly the period for which members remained on the funds, especially during periods of unemployment.

The subject of women's sickness experience in particular gave considerable anxiety to the departmental committee, and they made the following statement with regard to this difficult question:

Women's Sickness Experience.

"Taking women as a whole, experience shows that sufficient provision has not been made for the sickness benefit to women under the Act, that is, either the amount paid as premium is insufficient or the amount of the policy money is too great, and this applies both to single women and to married women.

"This fact is masked in the cases of certain societies by segregation, and in the case of other societies is intensified by segregation.

"The sickness claims of women have presented special difficulties by reason also of (*a*) the greater difficulty of determining the question of incapacity in the case of women, and (*b*) the inexperience in the conduct of women's insurance of those administering the societies."

As time went by the increasing difficulties of providing against women's claims for sickness and disablement benefits gave rise to a series of enquiries, and the position is now more or less stabilised as the result of changes made in the Act of 1932. For an appreciation of the present position I would refer to the extract from the report of the fourth valuation set out in Appendix No. 5.

With regard to sickness visiting, the committee found that it was not carried out as efficiently as it might be for various reasons, amongst others because too often the visitor was a part-time, and not a full-time visitor, and because visits were not made before sickness benefit was paid. It was thought that the function of the sickness visitor was not generally understood, and they were sometimes required to give their opinion on medical matters, which could merely result in confusion.

Amongst the most important of the recommendations which were made in the departmental committee's report was that there should be established as soon as possible a system of medical referees, and that the appointments to this post should be made by the Commissioners.

The question of sickness visiting has continued to receive the close attention of the Ministry of Health from time to time, and it may be of interest to give an extract from the present edition of the Approved Societies' Handbook issued by that Department:

"The maintenance of an efficient system of sickness visitation is an essential part of the administration of a properly conducted society. The free use by a society of the services of Regional Medical Officers cannot in any way be regarded as a substitute for proper sickness visiting; these two methods of supervision are complementary to one another, and the effectiveness of one depends on there being adequate recourse to the other.

"A sick visitor should in no circumstances interfere with what is the doctor's province, e.g. by attempting to remove bandages, or by giving the patient instructions contrary to those of the doctor, or by urging him to declare off the funds and return to work without further reference by the insured person to his doctor. Inconsiderate action by a sick visitor may seriously prejudice a patient's progress towards recovery. Sick visitors should refrain from anything in the nature of criticism of the doctor's treatment which would be calculated to disturb the patient's confidence in his doctor.

" A society is not justified in accepting the sick visitor's opinion regarding capacity for work in a particular case as overriding that of the doctor attending the member, except in special circumstances where the information furnished as to the member's behaviour or activities is such as to be obviously inconsistent with incapacity. Where the sick visitor's report is such as to throw doubt upon the member's continued unfitness for work, notwithstanding that medical certificates are still submitted, the society's proper course is to refer the member for examination by a Regional Medical Officer.

" In arranging a service of sickness visiting, the following points should be borne in mind:—

" (*a*) A person selected for appointment as a sick visitor should be properly qualified for the specialised duties a visitor has to undertake; it is most undesirable that a pay steward or other local representative of a society should be empoyed for visiting. Moreover, sick visitors should be appointed by the committee of management and not by a local organisation.

" (*b*) As far as circumstances permit, sick visitors should be employed for whole time; but whether they are employed for whole or part time they should be remunerated on a salaried basis and not at a rate per visit paid."

For purposes incidental to the work of the Royal Commission on National Health Insurance the sickness and disablement experience in the years 1921-3 of a representative sample of the whole body of insured persons was analysed by the departmental actuarial committee set up by the Minister of Health on the recommendation of the Royal Commission; their report being published as an appendix to the report of the Commission. This analysis contained many disquieting features, and led to a much fuller examination of the whole problem by the Government Actuary, who reviewed the sickness and disablement experience of a group of societies for the period 1921-1927, and published this report in January 1930 (Cmd. 3548). From that report some extracts are made, and are set out hereunder. Following the issue of the report, at a later date, a memorandum was issued on the whole question of certification of incapacity for work by the Departments of Health (Memo.329—I.C.). In the course of that memorandum, a table[1] prepared by the Actuary is recast in rather a different fashion, and the following comparative statement of

Table given in Memo 329—I.C.

Comparative Statement of Benefit Experience in the years 1921-1927 (*rates of actual weeks of sickness to " expectation "*) *taking* 1921 *figures as* 100.

Year	Men.		Women			
			Unmarried		Married	
	Sickness Benefit	Disablement Benefit	Sickness Benefit	Disablement Benefit	Sickness Benefit	Disablement Benefit
1921 ..	100	100	100	100	100	100
1922 ..	117	120	121	112	130	111
1923 ..	113	133	125	128	146	136
1924 ..	128	150	144	143	175	158
1925 ..	129	154	153	165	192	189
1926 ..	142	172	153	185	197	221
1927 ..	141	185	160	198	206	259

benefit experience taking the 1921 figures as 100 brings out very much more clearly the disquieting character of the growth of the sickness benefit, and, still more serious, the disablement benefit. In Table A,[1] as the percentage of weeks of sickness to expectation is shown, it does not so clearly bring out the fact of the serious growth in the claims, the benefit in the case of men, both sickness and disablement, having for most of the years kept well inside the expectation. In the case of women the sickness benefit and the disablement benefit both increased substantially from a figure which was below the expectation to a figure much in excess of it.

The following extracts from the Actuary's memorandum are of interest:—

" The really significant fact is the growth in the number of claimants. In this respect the years 1921 and 1927 show the two extremes. Taking men, it is seen that, while 14 out of every 100 claimed sickness benefit in 1921, the proportion had grown to 23 in 1927. Among unmarried women the respective proportions

[1] Table A. See Appendix No. 6.

were 12 and 21, and among married women 19 and 38. The growth in the intervening years, though not regular, was practically continuous.

"A continuous growth in the number of persons claiming benefit has been experienced, and the increase is most pronounced, on the whole, in the claims of short duration.

"Of all claimants who passed from sickness benefit to disablement benefit in 1927, and ceased to draw benefit before the end of the year, more than one in six went off the funds almost immediately the benefit was reduced to the disablement rate. Within a month of the reduction 50 per cent. had been certified as capable of work, and within 8 weeks 70 per cent. had found their working capacity restored.

"... Since National Health Insurance was applied compulsorily to those who were in employment on July 15 1912, or who entered employment later, the insured population at the outset included no persons who were already disabled; cases of permanent invalidity among the insured would therefore begin at a very small number and would continuously increase until a stable condition was reached, and the insured population had accordingly become normally constituted from this point of view. The period during which the number of permanent invalids would accumulate was actuarially estimated at about ten years, and, while the disturbance of industrial conditions set up by the war may perhaps have resulted in its extension, it is improbable that it went on till 1927. In any case this factor, even if it were still operating in that year, would only serve to explain a moderate increase at the higher ages in the number of recipients of disablement benefit; it could not account fully for such increases as are shown from, say, aged 40 onwards."

In the Memorandum 329/I.C. issued by the Department attention was drawn to the fact that there had been in recent years "a rise in claims for sickness and disablement benefit so continuous in its operation and of such magnitude as to occasion grave concern among all engaged in the administration of these benefits."

It was pointed out that the general effect of a critical study of the facts ascertained by the Government Actuary's investigations is to create a strong presumption in favour of the view that the observed increase in claims has been due, in the main, to an increase in the number of persons who received sickness or disablement benefit though not incapable of work.

Consideration has been given, the Memorandum states, to three possible explanations of the great and continuous increase of claims for sickness and disablement benefit which has been observed since 1921—namely, (*a*) a great increase in incapacitating sickness, (*b*) a tendency of persons incapable of work who would not have claimed in earlier years to claim under present conditions, and (*c*) an increase in the number of claims, admitted for benefit, by persons who are not incapable of work. Of these, (*a*) is dismissed in the Memorandum because, first, there is no independent evidence of such a wide-spread deterioration of health of the insured population, and secondly, the explanation would be inconsistent with the internal evidence afforded by study of the distribution of the claims among different sections of the insured population. The explanation (*b*), although doubtless true to a limited extent, is quite inadequate as an explanation of the great increase that has been observed. The Departments are driven, therefore, to the conclusion that the main factor in the general increase of claims has been an increase in payments to persons who were not incapable of work.

The appointment of the regional medical staff of the Ministry, after the War, had been designed to give effect to the recommendations of the Departmental Committee of 1914 and the most striking statements in the memorandum 329—I.C. are those which deal with the comparison of results of references to the regional medical staff over the years 1922-1930. They are contained in the following extracts:

"The fact that cessation of benefit after reference is most frequent in the class whose claims had increased most between 1921 and 1927, and least in the class which showed the least increase in claims, tends to reinforce the belief that the increase in claims has been mainly an increase in claims by persons who were not incapable of work."

Evidence tending in the same direction is afforded by the following table, from which it appears that, while the number of references dealt with by the Regional Medical Staff has increased from about 130,000 in 1922 to 573,000 in the year 1930—a nearly fivefold increase—there has been no increase in the proportion of those referred who continued to draw benefit.

Year	Incapacity references dealt with* 000's		Percentage of persons referred continuing benefit	
	England and Wales	Scotland	England and Wales	Scotland
1922	114	16	40	44
1923	146	19	43	46
1924	184	21	42	44
1925	201	22	42	44
1926	377	41	39	39
1927	313	34	40	42
1928	399	38	38	41
1929	446	44	35	42
1930	531	42	34	45

* Reference to the year 1937 (see page 158) shews no improvement.

Had those who ceased to draw benefit represented those only about whose fitness for work there was room for a legitimate difference of medical opinion, together with those who might have regained their working capacity between the date of the last intermediate certificate issued prior to reference and the date when they ceased benefit after reference, it is difficult to believe that the great increase of references would not by now have been accompanied by a substantial increase in the proportion of those referred who were found to be incapable of work and continued to draw benefit after reference."

In drawing the attention of practitioners to the seriousness of the position the Department states:—

Statements (set out in the Memorandum) offered in explanation of the high proportion of insured persons on the lists of practitioners who, when referred, ceased benefit, support the general inference that, in cases sufficiently numerous to have an appreciable effect on the benefit funds, certificates are issued which are not in accordance with the doctor's considered opinion of his patient's capacity for work, but are based either on insufficient evidence of incapacity or on extraneous considerations which are quite irrelevant to the insured person's title to benefit under the National Health Insurance Act.

It is pointed out by the Department that it is nowhere suggested in this Memorandum that insurance practitioners as a whole have been responsible for the general result. On the contrary, the strongest evidence adduced respecting the issue of certificates of incapacity to persons who were not incapacitated is that derived from a comparison of the results of the work of different practitioners. In other words, the standard by which many are judged to have failed to exercise proper care in their issue of certificates is that afforded by comparison of the results of their work with that of a large number of their colleagues.

An examination of the statistics relating to sickness benefit discloses some interesting features which are rather difficult of explanation; for example, in England and Wales, although the amounts for 1925 and 1935 spent on sickness benefit correspond very closely, the amount being £9,300,000 in the first year and £9,100,000 in the later year, the cost of sickness benefit varied between the years 1921 and 1935 as widely as £7,000,000 in 1921, and £12,000,000 in 1929. It must be presumed that the very high rate of sickness benefit which was reached in 1929, and the publication of the Government Actuary's review of sickness experience from 1921-27, did result in something of a shock to the Approved Societies and the medical profession, and that the decline which has been witnessed since the peak figure of 1929 was reached must be attributed to some extent to the special attention which has been given to this matter by all the parties concerned.

Chapter VIII

Insurance and National Providence

(*a*) *The general success of compulsory insurance.*

The Royal Commission's report is very definite in its expressions of satisfaction at the general success of the scheme of compulsory health insurance, e.g. (page 16):—

"We are satisfied that the scheme of National Health Insurance has fully justified itself and has, on the whole, been successful in operation. The workers of this country have obtained under it substantial advantages, in particular by securing the title to free medical attention and medicine whenever and as soon as these are required, and by the proportionate diminution, to the extent of the cash benefit granted, of their anxiety as to the loss of wages during illness. Furthermore, the scheme has, on the whole, been satisfactorily administered, notwithstanding the difficulties and antagonisms at the outset, and the peculiar and urgent problems which arose when vast numbers of men left insurable employment for the theatres of war and their place in the industries of the country was taken by women entering insurance, consequently, for the first time. The contributions have been collected and the benefits provided with a marked degree of efficiency. We are convinced that National Health Insurance has now become a permanent feature of the social system of this country, and should be continued on its present compulsory and contributory basis."

And again (page 14):

"We have had little criticism of the scope of the scheme so far as concerns the persons included in it. Most of the witnesses were, moreover, practically at one in their approval of the present method of deriving the revenue, that is to say, by means of compulsory contributions from employers and workers with a proportionate contribution from the National Exchequer; though it may be observed that the National Confederation of Employers' Organisations pressed strongly for a reduction of the contribution and the assignment of a larger proportion of the cost than hitherto to the State."

Though satisfied as to the general success of the scheme, the Royal Commission is in no doubt that changes, however drastic and far-reaching, may have to be made, sooner or later (page 116):

"We hold that the National Health Insurance scheme was in the nature of a great and novel experiment in the field of social welfare, and that it must now be open to Parliament, untrammelled and unfettered, to review the whole scheme in the light of thirteen years' experience of its working and to make such changes, however drastic, as that experience may have shown to be desirable."

I have dealt elsewhere with the case for the continuation of a scheme administered by the present machinery. On the question of the arguments for a different scheme, the Report says (page 117):

"The scheme of Health Insurance contemplated in 1911 was only a national scheme in the sense that the State undertook to enforce the payment of contributions in respect of those to whom the Act applied. It was thus a State scheme which relied for its fulfilment on voluntary effort, and which in intention was careful to make the utmost use of voluntary and competing organisations already in the field. On a survey of the present position it may appear to some arguable that a different scheme should be established now, but it is not, we think, permissible to base such an argument on a supposed conflict between the 'national' promise of 1911, and the subsequent failure to realise these earlier ideals."

As to extensions which are immediately practicable, the Commissioners (page 73) make the definite recommendation that only such extensions or modifications as involve no expenditure, or can be met within the present financial resources of the scheme, should be considered as immediately practicable. "This implies that, in our opinion, there should be no increase at the present time in the rates of contribution under the scheme. We consider also that the scheme should be self-supporting subject to the payment by the Exchequer of its present proportionate share of the cost of benefits and their administration, together with the cost of the general supervision of the scheme by the Ministry of Health and the Scottish Board of Health. We recommend that beyond these charges no further liability should rest on the Exchequer in any circumstances."

The possibility of making provision under the present scheme for a considerable section of the population who seriously need provision by way of insurance but who are not under contract of service and, therefore, do not come within the provisions of the scheme for employed contributors, appears to have been examined by the Royal Commission and disposed of rather lightly as impracticable. It may be agreed at once that as regards a mere extension of the present scheme the opportunities for development seemed somewhat remote, but in this, as in other respects to which I shall make a further reference, I cannot help feeling that the Royal Commission rather missed an opportunity. It may be that, in a sense, as Professor Gray and Sir Andrew Duncan say, in the course of a statement which I shall quote presently, the subject of co-ordinating the various schemes of social insurance was outside the scope of the Royal Commission, and it is equally certain that within the definite terms of their reference they had quite enough to do to report upon the scheme of National Health Insurance in all its detail. But when the question of co-ordinating the various insurance and pension services come to be tackled, as it must be very soon, then I am quite sure that this question of the workers who are not within the provisions of compulsory insurance at present has got to be faced and the problem settled. The actual terms in which the Royal Commission's report refers to this matter are as follows:—

(P.200) "We have considered whether it is possible and desirable to make provision for the voluntary insurance of the small shop-keeper, the hawker, the crofter, and the like. We questioned Sir Walter Kinnear on this subject and may quote from his reply: 'There is, of course, no employer of such persons, so that there is no machinery by which we could properly get in the contributions. The Commission are aware that the 1911 Act allowed such persons to be insured as voluntary contributors at a rate of contribution graded according to their ages. The Ryan Committee in 1916 recommended that admission to this class should be abolished on the ground that only some 28,000 persons had availed themselves of the right of voluntary insurance and this number did not justify the troublesome administrative machinery that was required. This was done by the 1918 Act. Under the Contributory Pensions Act passed during this year a very wide door has been opened for a limited time to entry into voluntary insurance of persons who have at some time since July, 1912, had 104 weeks' insurance or excepted employment. So that, of course, the matter to a large extent has rectified itself. This will meet the case of the great majority of persons not now insured who may reasonably be allowed into voluntary insurance. It would not be practicable without a grading of contributions to give a continuing right to uninsured persons to come in as voluntary contributors, and we rather suggest that no extension of the existing provisions in this respect is called for, especially in view of the Pensions Act of this year.' "

The real question which has sooner or later to be faced with regard to the very considerable section of the community of like economic status with the "employed" is not that of voluntary but compulsory insurance.

There is one other general matter to which I may refer in this conclusion of the review of the insurance as distinct from the health aspects of the enquiry which is the subject of this book. The whole of the funds collected under the insurance scheme, whether from employers or employed, together with the State contribution paid towards benefit, become virtually the funds of the Approved Societies, and are administered by them. It is true that, as we have noted, the administration of the funds of the Approved Societies is subject to a very tight control on the part of the central department, and it may be, therefore, that the point which I am about to make has not quite so much force as it otherwise would have. The fact is that employers who contribute about one-third of the total sum have no share in the administration of the scheme. This question is glanced at in the following extract from the report of the Royal Commission, which deals with a matter which is rather fully examined in Appendix No. 4, to which reference is made elsewhere. The extract relates to the question of the setting free of some parts of the future surpluses of the Approved Societies for the purpose of financing, in supplementation of the margin which was found to exist in the contribution, certain developments of the service which were recommended in the report of the Commission. (In passing it may be noted that these developments did not materialise).

(p. 121): "The proportion of this surplus which should be brought into the pool would clearly have to be substantial, since otherwise the pooling scheme would be ineffective. On the other hand the proportion left with the societies would also have to be substantial if the incentive to good administration is not to be weakened. Our conclusion, therefore, is that the proportion should be one-half, a proportion which could also be defended on the ground that one-half of the contributions out of which the surplus arises is paid not by the members themselves but by their employers. The pooling of one-half of the surplus acquired would have the same effect broadly as if the employers' contributions were carried to a central fund and one-half of all the benefits and other charges paid thereout —a plan which might with some measure of justification have been adopted from the beginning."

(*b*) *The Trend towards a Ministry of Social Insurance.*

I have ventured to set down certain broad general conclusions with regard to the Insurance and Provident aspects of my subject; in a later chapter I record certain provisional conclusions on the Health problem, reserving in that case the right to modify those conclusions as the result of the more complete and detailed examination of the subject which is essential.

The National Health Insurance scheme has brought about some very definite achievements. In conjunction with unemployment insurance it has established the acceptance of the compulsory principle by the employer and the employed person. The scheme has brought a very large measure of insurance under the control of the central government and it has led to the appointment of a Government Actuary, who is now available for advising the central government with regard to the financial soundness of many far reaching schemes in the great field of social expenditure, which has grown tenfold within the last quarter of a century. Although as regards a great deal of this expenditure the matter may be outside his province, it is at any rate a great achievement to have an actuary who first of all advised upon the problems which arose in connexion with National Health Insurance, and then emerged as the Government Actuary whose function it is to advise in a great many other fields of activity.

We have seen how through the ages the main desire of the citizen in the field of providence has been to see that there should be money forthcoming for a decent burial or funeral and, by whatever name you may choose to call it, there is to be found in this form of provision the beginnings of the present system of insurance. We have seen also how the old friendly societies had their foundations in social or convivial gatherings, how there emerged from these a communal desire to provide for sickness and a decent burial, and how the old social gathering and the old club night or lodge meeting have gradually lost a great deal of their attraction. When the National Health Insurance scheme came on the scene we were all fully intent on making use of the existing organisations, and it seemed proper to record in the statute that every society undertaking the new scheme must be under the definite control of its members. Whatever may be said with regard to the old friendly societies, the fact is that when the insurance companies and the collecting societies came on the scene and took such a considerable part in the administration of the new insurance scheme, the prospects of government by the members became very small indeed, but with our usual fondness for make-believe it is preserved on the statute book. Frankly, however, this does not matter very much; what really matters is that we were able to take what was already in existence and use it as the machinery for bringing into operation an enormous scheme of compulsory health insurance; what matters also is that this vast machine came under the control of the central government. In the course of administration a host of officials—secretaries and others—have become well versed in administration, and we have a large trained body of men who do the job probably quite as well as government servants or servants of local authorities—some may say a good deal better. Even with regard to the surpluses disclosed on valuation, which are presumed to be created to a large extent by the good government of the separate societies, the stern figures of the Minister of Health and the Government Actuary are there all the time to prevent the societies "playing ducks and drakes" with what they have been taught to regard as their own money.

While the friendly societies, with what is left of the old friendly society spirit, have managed to maintain a fairly steady flow of members and to keep up their membership in the aggregate, we have seen how there has been a falling away from those societies where the members are supposed to turn up on lodge nights and keep a watchful eye on events, and a considerable increase on the other hand in those societies, the deposit and dividing societies, where the element of provision for the family as distinct from self-interest is, shall we say, not quite so evident. Outside the compulsory provisions of the National Health Insurance scheme, the developments and the drive are to be found amongst the deposit and dividing societies, the collecting companies and the insurance companies. Examination of the figures available[1] does not encourage the idea that there has been any very considerable growth amongst the working classes of real and substantial provision for dependants as distinct from the old idea of provision for a decent burial. Progress there has undoubtedly been, but in the absence of detailed information with regard to the sort of progress which has been made, it would seem that the amount of provision made for dependants amongst the working classes generally does not appear to be of any appreciable magnitude; putting by for a rainy day is the predominant element, but coupled to a large extent with a desire to provide for dependants as in the case of "endowment" insurance.

Running side by side with the National Health Insurance scheme we have, of course, the scheme for contributory pensions administered by the central department—in England the Ministry of Health and the non-contributory old age pension administered by the same department; and the vast commitments of the Government in regard to unemployment, both under the Unemployment Insurance scheme and the Unemployment Assistance scheme, the latter, of course, being not an insurance provision at all, but definite State assistance, taking the place of a good deal of the relief which was administered under the old poor law.

The anomalies arising from the separate machinery of the Unemployment and Health Insurance schemes were fully present to the minds of the Royal Commission, as shown by the two following extracts, and it may be noted in passing that when the Commission state that both schemes are designed to alleviate the distress arising from the cessation of income due to causes beyond the workers' control this applies equally to the various provisions for pensions, which are now in existence. I give a third extract,

[1] Reference may be made to the figures given at the end of appendix No. 2 showing that the average sum assured for each whole life policy in 1935 was £15 only, and that the average sum per policy of endowment assurance was £26 only. The figures which are given in that estimate as to the number of policies taken out are so vastly in excess of the total population that it is clear that several policies are taken out in respect of each life, and therefore it is impossible to estimate what is the average amount for which one life is assured.

from the "reservations" contained in the separate statement in the Report appended to the Report, written by Sir Andrew Duncan and Professor Alexander Gray, and it seems to me that in this place only is the importance of the far-reaching problem which has to be tackled, properly recognised.

(p.139): "The need for financial help must in general be greater in a period of ill-health than in a period of unemployment of the same duration. The existing position seems to us difficult to defend. Differences of machinery, such as the Employment Exchange system in the one case and the Approved Society system in the other, a single fund in the one and segregated funds in the other, can be justified. But here we are concerned with the actual provision made in the homes of those who are in closely similar circumstances of distress."

(p.26): "We may be permitted to refer to certain disparities between the Health and the Unemployment Insurance Schemes. In the latter the standard rate of benefit is 18/- a week, and additions of 5/- are made for the wife and 2/- for each dependent child. It is difficult, in our opinion, to justify a less generous provision for the invalid than for the man in good health, whose circumstances certainly involve smaller expenditure. It is equally difficult to justify the existence of two State schemes side by side, one of which recognises the needs of dependants and the other does not, in circumstances of hardship closely similar. Both schemes are designed to alleviate the distress arising from the cessation of income due to causes beyond the worker's control, and the question whether these causes are to be sought in ill-health or in the failure of employment has no bearing on the needs of dependants.

"It has been suggested to us by the National Association of Trade Union Approved Societies that, as a consequence of the higher rate of unemployment benefit there may be a temptation to apply for that benefit rather than for sickness benefit, even though the applicant may be incapable of work, and so fulfil the statutory condition for the latter. In such a case he would, of course, be really disentitled to receive unemployment benefit. We have received no direct evidence on the point and, in any case, such evidence would probably be difficult to obtain. We do not doubt that this question, which primarily affects the administration of Unemployment Insurance, is fully in the minds of the officials of the Ministry of Labour."

Here is the extract from the Duncan and Gray "reservations":

(p.292): "The first point to which we wish to draw attention—the lack of co-ordination in our social services—is one which has been the subject of comment in many quarters. We desire in this place to point out the inconvenience, and by implication the waste which it occasions. It would be unjust to say that our social legislation has grown up haphazard, but it is indubitable that the various schemes contrived for the protection of the worker against the accidents of life have been elaborated—doubtless very properly—as and when occasion offered. Poor Law Relief, Old Age Pensions, Health Insurance, Unemployment Insurance, Widows' Pensions have grown up in large measure independently: When they are reviewed, they are reviewed independently. They are financed in different ways; they are operated by different agencies. On the possibility of co-ordination, on the alternative methods and machinery of operating a co-ordinated scheme, we have received no evidence, or only incidental evidence; and on all such matters we express no opinion. But we do desire to emphasise that there is here a problem which calls for urgent consideration. It may be that in a co-ordinated scheme different machinery would still be necessary for the administration of different sections of the work undertaken, but *prima facie* it appears reasonable to assume that an economy of expenditure and of effort would be effected by viewing the problem of social insurance as a whole and not sectionally."

In the few observations which I make in conclusion of the whole of the examination of this subject of insurance, as distinct from health, I would like to say that I am fully conscious of the need for caution in coming too readily to the conclusion that, because subjects are labelled "insurance," they are suitable for merging under one scheme, or under one central department. But at the same time no one will question that, as stated by Duncan and Gray, the problem is one which calls for urgent consideration. If reference is made to the total annual expenditure on those social services which are insurance or pensions, as set out in the statement at page 96, it will be seen that there is a very vast expenditure here amounting to £260,000,000, which is the subject of many different administrations, and it does really appear, without being dogmatic on the subject, that within this vast total expenditure there is scope for co-ordination, for economies, and for developments; developments, it may be noted, which would be possible within the total amount of the present expenditure.

The question therefore arises whether there should not be established a Ministry of Social Insurance under which the various forms of statutory provision for insurance against sickness, old age, and unemployment would be securely established, and developed, not only as regards the workers of this country but as regards the body corporate as a whole. The care which is bestowed on the provision for the employed persons in this country, using the expression "the employed" in the sense in which it has been defined in the Insurance Acts, must be due in large measure to the importance of keeping the economic machine well-oiled, and also undoubtedly to the fact that it is so convenient to collect the contributions by means of deduction from wages. But there is a large body of persons outside the ranks of the so-called "employed" persons who are left to make whatever provision they think fit by a means of voluntary insurance. Under the National Health Insurance scheme, voluntary insurance at the outset was a dismal failure, and although there has been a certain revival in recent years amongst former "employed contributors," owing to the fact that old age pensions are now included in the provision, it is equally true that the expansion of voluntary insurance since the pension was added has not all been amongst those persons for whom the provision was intended.

Marriage is still a fundamental institution of society, and although possibly it has since the beginning of the century received a considerable number of hard blows and by some would be said to be shaking on its foundations, the family is still the recognised social unit. It is surely not too much to say that provision for disability and old age and for dependants should be made compulsory, just as the payment of rates and taxes is compulsory, and that such provision by way of compulsory insurance should be organised in due course under a Ministry of Social Insurance, to proceed along well-ordered definite lines of development, with the aim that the main responsibility of the public authority would tend to become the control of insurance provision designed to avert as far as possible the onset of distress, rather than the relief of distress which has arrived.

P.S. TO CHAPTER VIII—AUGUST 1945

The unification of the various schemes of social insurance foreshadowed in this chapter is about to become an accomplished fact.

A Minister of National Insurance has been appointed. The powers and functions of his Ministry and the scope of the proposals for the amalgamation and extension of the various schemes of insurance will, it is anticipated, be the subject of early legislation in the new Parliament. It can safely be assumed, in view of the universal acceptance of the proposals in the Beveridge Report, that the main recommendations of that report will be followed in broad outline. They include the following:—

Unification of social insurance in respect of contributions, enabling each insured person to obtain all benefits by a single weekly contribution on a single document.

Unification of social insurance and assistance, in respect of administration, in a Ministry of Social Security with local Security Offices within reach of all insured persons.

Supersession of the present system of Approved Societies.

Supersession of the present scheme of workmen's compensation and inclusion of provision for industrial accident or disease within the unified social insurance scheme.

Separation of medical treatment from the administration of cash benefits and the setting up of a comprehensive medical service for every citizen, covering all treatment and every form of disability under the supervison of the Health Departments.

Extension of insurance against prolonged disability to all persons gainfully occupied and of insurance for retirement pensions to all persons of working age, whether gainfully occupied or not.

Assimilation of benefit and pension rates for unemployment, disability, other than prolonged disability due to industrial accident or disease, and retirement.

Assimilation of contribution conditions for unemployment and disability benefit, except where disability is due to industrial accident or disease, and revision of contribution conditions for pension.

Abolition of the exceptions from insurance.

Inclusion of universal funeral grant in compulsory insurance.

Transfer to the Ministry of Social Security of the remaining functions of Local Authorities in respect of public assistance, other than treatment and services of an institutional character.

Transfer to the Ministry of Social Security of the functions of the Assistance Board, of the work of the Customs and Excise Department in respect of non-contributory pensions, and probably of the employment service of the Ministry of Labour and National Service, in addition to unemployment insurance, and the work of other departments in connection with the administration of cash benefits of all kinds, including workmen's compensation.

PART II
NATIONAL HEALTH

PART II—NATIONAL HEALTH

Introductory Note (1938).

It had been my purpose when I started on this investigation to devote the main part of the paper to an examination of the question of the contribution which the insurance medical service has made or is making towards the realisation of an organised health service for the community, but I have had to alter my conception of the present scope of the research and limit this part of the paper, in the main, to an examination of the foundations, the content, and the general trend of the insurance medical service.

It was important, of course, that the medical benefit provisions should be effectively designed as a part of the machinery for the provision of cash benefits, but a question of machinery is of minor importance compared with that of the relation of the problem to the whole question of the public health. Those who think that it is vital for the medical benefit provisions to be associated with the insurance machinery, and that the insurance machine should control the medical profession, do not perhaps have sufficient regard to the fact that the doctor's first concern must be the welfare of his patient, and that no other considerations should stand in the way of the honest exercise of his primary duty. If Health should become the function of one central authority, and Insurance that of another, certification could always be arranged between the two central administering authorities, and controlled more effectively by the central health authority than by the central insurance authority.

There has appeared, while I have been engaged upon this study, the Report on the British Health Services issued by P.E.P. from their offices, 16, Queen Anne's Gate, S.W.1. An examination of this report has satisfied me that it would be quite impracticable, within the limited scope of what has become part II of the present paper, to make an adequate contribution to the question of the organisation of the medical services of the country.

The PEP publication is prefaced by an introductory note in which it is stated that the survey of the British Health services has proved one of the most complex and difficult tasks yet undertaken by PEP. The subject, it is said, suffers from a bewildering number of fragmentary and often conflicting specialisms, medical, administrative, and financial. As an indication of the amount of correspondence and labour involved, and of the co-operation which the group has been fortunate enough to secure in its task, it is mentioned that more than two hundred different persons and organisations have supplied material or revised drafts for various sections of the report. And notwithstanding this, the report concludes with the following statement. " The type of survey, as we have attempted it, should be carried out much more thoroughly as an essential and continuous function of government. There should be men and women constantly tracing back into the factory, the office, the traffic system, and the home, the origins of defects and diseases which are a burden on the nation."

In the light of such a statement, one investigator may well be deterred from attempting anything in the shape of an effective contribution towards the question of an organised medical service. I think, however, that I should set out a short list of books and publications of which I have already made some study, and confine myself in the main to references in these publications which have a more immediate bearing on the question of the insurance medical service. They are as follows :—

Medical Benefit. A study of the experience of Germany and Denmark—Gibbon —published by P. S. King & Sons 1912.

The Battle of the Clubs. A reprint of the reports of the special Commissioner of *The Lancet* published in London at the offices of *The Lancet.* (1896).

An Investigation into the Economic Conditions of Contract Medical Practice in the United Kingdom : published by the British Medical Association, 1905.

National Health Insurance and the Medical Profession : by Dr. Hoffman, published by the Prudential Press of Newark, U.S.A. 1920. (In addition to this American publication I have read a great many pamphlets, mostly very critical of the National Health Insurance scheme published by the American Medical Association from time to time).

Proposals for a General Medical Service for the Nation : published by the B.M.A., August 1930, and in a revised form in April, 1938.

Patient and Doctor : by Sir Henry Brackenbury, Hodder and Stoughton, 1935.

Medicine and the State : Sir Arthur Newsholme, George Allen and Unwin Ltd. 1932.

The Report of the Consultative Council on Medical and Allied Services on the subject of the future provision of medical allied services, published in 1920 by the Stationery Office. Cmd. 693.

The Report of the Committee on Scottish Health Services 1936. Cmd. 5204.

A convenient summary of the provisions of the several National Sickness Insurance systems is contained in a pamphlet issued by the American Medical Association at Chicago, entitled "Sickness Insurance and Sickness Costs." (See also the references at the beginning of chapter II).

Addendum (1945)

If the publication of the P.E.P. survey deterred this writer from embarking upon any further review of the health services, the publication of the Beveridge report, and the issue of the Government White Paper in 1943 have rendered such a review a work of supererogation. Part II of this Enquiry into National Health Insurance therefore stands as it was written, with the necessary textual revision, and the new chapter 16 gives a sufficient summary of the White Paper proposals and of the progress of the discussions between the medical profession and the Government.

Chapter IX

The Insurance Medical Service described

Introductory Note.

Dr. Hoffman, in his critical examination of the question of the relations of the National Health Insurance and the medical profession, gives a long schedule of publications which at that time had already been issued by the Insurance Acts Committee of the British Medical Association, which is admittedly the body recognised as representative of the whole insurance medical profession. Dr. Hoffman says that these publications are but a fragment of a truly enormous literature which has never been subjected to critical examination by those familiar with the facts of actual experience. Such a task, he says, "is now practically beyond the power of any one man or even of a group of men, officially occupied as they would be with the flood of current reports, rules, regulations, circulars, etc., frequently effecting profound changes in matters of law and procedure."

Notwithstanding Dr. Hoffman's view the volume of "Medical Insurance Practice," by R. W. Harris and Leonard Shoeten Sack, published by the British Medical Association, and in possession of most of the doctors engaged in insurance practice, the fourth edition of which appeared in January 1937, does serve as a complete and fully indexed work of reference to the medical benefit provisions of the National Health Insurance Act and to the "flood" of rules and circulars and may be consulted by any reader who wishes to understand in detail what the working of the medical insurance scheme involves.

Within the limits of this present paper it is only possible to refer to the essentials in the scheme, and to examine the working of the scheme on broad lines. Medical practitioners in 1911 were confronted with service under a scheme which represented to most of them a veritable revolution in the conditions of medical service. Notwithstanding this, the chosen leaders of the profession, the British Medical Association, sufficiently appreciated the fact that the new system would provide for the medical treatment of the whole "employed" population under conditions which, both for doctor and patient, were greatly superior to the conditions of contract practice under which a substantial section of the working population had hitherto been treated. It was, therefore, worth while to make the new scheme work if certain cardinal points could be secured. They accordingly imposed certain conditions under which the medical profession would undertake to work the new Act—conditions designed as far as possible to preserve in a national service as many as possible of the features of private practice, and to ensure that in the new national service the medical profession had as large a share as possible in the guidance, if not the control, of the administrative machine. It must be fairly admitted that in both respects the scheme secures to the medical profession all that can reasonably be expected, and that on every occasion when amendments have been made the advice and assistance of the body representative of the medical profession has been sought at every stage and the profession given an increasing share in the administration.

That the new service made a bad start has to be recorded. During the final stages of the passage of the Bill through Parliament and immediately it became law, the prospect of the new medical service being still-born became a serious menace owing to the stubborn resistance of the medical profession to the proposed rate of remuneration. The opposition persisted in an aggravated form down to the end of the year 1912 when the service was due to begin. The funds available for the service were demonstrably ample for an effective and well-paid salaried service ; possibly the knowledge of this, and of the fact that the extra

Exchequer grant which had been offered was known to represent the limit to which the Government was prepared to go, combined to bring about a collapse of the opposition of the medical profession at the eleventh hour. The doctors signed the agreements for service almost precipitately, and everywhere, with a few negligible exceptions, where the difficulties were surmounted after a short interval, a full and effective service was secured.

Before proceeding to give a description of the principal features of the medical service for the insured, I give one or two extracts from the late Sir Henry Brackenbury's book. He wrote with unquestioned and unique authority to deal with the subject:—

"The National Insurance Act was passed in 1911, and the system of medical benefit under that Act came into force in January 1913. The system, even within the area it was intended to cover, had many imperfections, and still has some. It is extraordinarily complicated in its machinery, but by the united efforts of the Government Departments concerned, of the local Insurance Committees, of the Approved Societies, and of the organised medical profession, the major defects have been overcome, and the system may now be said to be working effectively, though simplification and adjustments are still required. Some nine years ago the Representative Body of the British Medical Association, almost without dissent, declared that 'the measure of success which has attended the experiment of providing medical benefit under the National Health Insurance Acts has been sufficient to justify the profession in uniting to secure the continuance and improvement of an insurance system.' Since then further resolutions have been adopted pressing for an extension of the system to bodies of persons who are not at present included in it, and by a growing conviction, born of the intimate experience of twenty-two years, it is acknowledged that any suggestion of the abolition of the system would be received by an overwhelming and emphatic protest from the medical profession and insured population alike. The Association, in its evidence before the Royal Commission on National Health Insurance, enumerated thus the benefits of the system: "(*a*) Large numbers, indeed whole classes, of persons are now receiving a real medical attention which they formerly did not receive at all; (*b*) the number of practitioners in proportion to the population in densely populated areas has increased; (*c*) the amount and character of the medical attention is immensely superior to that formerly given in the great majority of clubs; (*d*) illness is now coming under skilled observation and treatment at an earlier stage than was formerly the case; (*e*) the work of practitioners has been given a bias towards prevention that was formerly not so marked; (*f*) clinical records are being provided which may be made of great service in relation to public health and medical research; (*g*) co-operation among practitioners is being encouraged to an increasing degree; (*h*) there is now more marked recognition than formerly of the collective responsibility of the profession to the community in respect of all health matters."

"It might have been added," says Brackenbury, "that in a number of rural areas it has been found possible to maintain medical attention in places which would otherwise have been left derelict."

And here is another extract from his book:

"There are three particular features of the British system of national insurance which are extremely valuable. These are: (1) every registered medical practitioner has a right to be a member of the service; (2) the conditions of the service as between patient and doctor approximate closely to those which obtain in private practice; (3) the medical profession is assigned a considerable share in the administration. No lay body can select the doctors who shall be allowed to serve and exclude others from serving, except in so far as serious neglect of duty may be proved against any doctor actually serving. Thus the patient has a very wide choice from among all those doctors who elect to make their services available. Because of, not in spite of, the confidence in the profession which these three features disclose, provision has to be made for the occasional delinquent. If the State has no right to appoint selected doctors to take part in the service, machinery has to be established for dealing with any one who conspicuously fails in his duty. If the State has limited its function to bringing together doctor and patient, leaving them free thereafter to act in accordance with recognised or traditional methods, it must provide means whereby, in case of dispute, each may be sure of a square deal. If the State leaves purely medical matters to be judged by a purely professional body, there must be some authoritative delimitation of the respective spheres. There have to be, therefore, a considerable number of rules or regulations, but in fact these need not trouble the doctor any more than the ordinary requirements of the penal code trouble the law-abiding citizen."

The following are the essential features of the insurance medical service:

(1) The service is a general practitioner service (excluding confinements).

(2) Every insured person (which means the great majority of employed persons) is entitled to the service wherever he may be in Great Britain.

(3) Every qualified medical practioner is entitled to put his name on the medical list and to take part in the service.

(4) Free choice of doctor by patient and of patient by doctor.

(5) The dispensing of prescriptions by pharmacists.

(6) The issue of certificates of incapacity for work to enable the insured person to draw cash payments during illness.

(7) The payment of the doctor by a quarterly cheque representing a capitation fee for each insured person on his list, well or ill; consequently no fee-charging or account-keeping.

(8) Central and local administrative control; with the medical profession closely consulted and given a share in the various branches of the administration.

The care of his patient must be the doctor's first consideration; this is equally true of private practice and practice under an insurance system. It is also to the doctor's interest under the insurance system; critics of the system commonly overlook the fact that a doctor who is paid by a capitation fee for every person on his list, whether well or ill, has a real inducement to keep his patients well.

As the care of the patient is an individual doctor's first responsibility, so it must be the concern of the National Insurance scheme to secure for every insured person, wherever he may be in the country in which the scheme is the law of the land, immediate medical attention when he requires it; and the National Health Insurance scheme is so designed. Every insured person, while he remains insured (and this covers considerable periods when there are unpaid contributions owing to sickness and unemployment) is entitled to medical benefit. The sole qualification is the fact that he is insured. The doctors collectively have a responsibility for the treatment of the whole insured population. This is effected in the following way:

> An insured person is entitled to select as his regular medical attendant, from a list (or panel) of doctors in the area who have undertaken insurance practice, any doctor who is willing to put him on his list. There is thus free choice of doctor by the patient and of patient by the doctor. If the doctor to whom application is made is not willing to accept the insured person on his permanent list, he has to give hm such treatment as is immediately required and advise him of the steps necessary to secure his being placed on some other doctor's list; if an insured person has been refused acceptance he must not be left in doubt as to what to do next. If, therefore, he is not accepted by a doctor—an unlikely contingency—he may be assigned to some doctor by the local authority, the Insurance Committee. Further, when the insured person is on a doctor's list, he must not be left without treatment if his own doctor is not available, and the scheme, therefore, provides for treatment to be given by any insurance practitioner in an emergency or when the insured person is staying away from home. The practitioner is entitled to require the insured person to produce the medical card —which is issued to every insured person and which, therefore, ought to be in his possession—either as proof of his identity if he claims to be on that practitioner's list or, if he is not, as evidence of his title to benefit. When the doctor is in doubt as to the title to benefit of the person who represents that he is an insured person, he is required to give any necessary treatment and may charge by way of returnable deposit a reasonable fee, giving a special form of receipt to the patient to enable him to claim repayment. Payment for the treatment of another doctor's patients in any emergency or when away from home is provided for by machinery which need not be described here.

Change of doctor.

With regard to free choice of doctor, the system at first in force provided that a change within the same district could only be effected at the end of each half-year. This was abandoned after some years as unsatisfactory in favour of a system which provided for unrestricted change of doctor at any time, and this after fair trial was in turn replaced by a system which secures that an immediate change may be made at any time with the consent of the two doctors concerned, but that, failing such consent, an insured person may only change his doctor at the end of a quarter.

In general, it may be said that the present arrangement works very well; on the one hand a patient does not remain unfairly tied to a doctor in whom he has lost confidence, and on the other hand there is a sufficient check on impulsive change and on that sort of turnover to another doctor which has for its motive a desire for easier certification.

The improper charging of fees.

The question of fee charging is a cause of stumbling to many doctors who do not wish to be imposed upon or are perhaps a little over-anxious that they shall not render any services for which they are not paid. A doctor must not demand or accept any payment in respect of the treatment which he is required to give to any person who is on his list or who represents that he is an insured person, except as already stated, by way of deposit in cases of doubt. It is for the applicant to represent that he is an insured person, but the wise doctor will always put this question "beyond a peradventure," e.g., by asking the nature of the person's employment. Some misguided insured persons will insist upon treatment as private patients, and, when a doctor so treats for a fee an insured person who is not in fact on his list, he is not committing a technical breach of his terms of service. But it is hardly necessary to say that the frequent treatment of insured persons as private patients is bound to have unfortunate reactions on the good name of the service and to prejudice the position of the doctor concerned. If an insured person clearly understands from his doctor that there will be no difference in the kind of treatment that he will receive, whether he is treated as a private patient or as an insured person, and that his doctor is already paid by way of insurance premium, he is hardly likely to want to make a fresh payment when he falls ill. Seeing that doctors as a general rule take a wide and generous view of their collective responsibility for the treatment of the insured population, it is possible to add without offence that what may be called "fee-snatching," in so far as the doctor just keeps within the letter of his agreement, is at least open to the charge of meanness and, when the agreement is broken, constitutes an offence which is properly regarded as a serious one, bringing discredit on the service.

The definition of duties in the agreement.

The terms of the doctor's agreement, which are embodied in regulations made by the Minister of Health, define the persons for whose treatment the practitioner is responsible, and the evidence of the person's title to obtain treatment; and to these reference has already been made. The range of service which is to be given is defined as "all proper and necessary medical services other than those involving the application of skill and experience of a degree or kind which general practitioners as a class cannot reasonably be expected to possesss." In other words, the service is a general practitioner service—with the important exception that confinements, but not ante-natal care, are excluded. If it is claimed by a practitioner that the service which he renders demands special skill and experience the onus is laid upon him of proving that he possesses such skill and experience, and that the operation or other service is outside the above definition. When these questions are raised by an insurance practitioner, they are, under regulations, settled in the first place by his medical colleagues in the area and may be sent ultimately to special referees.

A practitioner's general duties towards his patients comprise attendance at his surgery at his registered hours, which must provide satisfactory facilities; the provision of proper and sufficient surgery and waiting room accommodation; an obligation to "visit and treat a patient whose condition so requires" at any place within the district in which the practitioner has undertaken to visit patients; the issue of medical certificates free of charge in accordance with the rules; the writing and in some cases the dispensing of prescriptions for drugs and appliances; the keeping of records of treatment of his patients; the making of reports to medical officers of the Ministry where the doctor's certificate of incapacity for work has been called in question; and various other matters. The conditions under which deputies, assistants, or partners may be employed, while the overriding responsibility of the practitioner himself is preserved, are all carefully set out in the regulations. The provisions will all be found on closer examination to be such as may reasonably be looked for in any scheme of this kind, and, within my own experience, are sufficiently elastic in their operation.

I have reserved for a somewhat fuller examination in two succeeding chapters the question of the practitioner s remuneration, and three important questions of machinery—certificates, prescriptions, and records.

The local administration.

The medical profession having, as already noted, refused to carry out their duties under the control of the approved societies, it became necessary to create new local authorities, called insurance committees, for each county or county borough. The insurance committee is a body varying in size from 20 to 40 members; three fifths of the committee's members represent insured persons and one-fifth are appointed by the county or the county borough council. Of the council's nominees one or two must be women. Representation of the medical profession is provided for, and the remaining members (from one to four) consist of chemists or women members appointed by the Minister.

The establishment of these insurance committees was in the nature of a compromise removing the doctors from the direct control of the societies and at the same time preserving in each committee a majority representation for the approved societies which, as we have seen, are assumed to be under the control of their members.

From long personal experience I am satisfied that these representatives of insured persons, whether officials of Approved Societies or members of the executives of the societies, do take a very real interest in the question of the effective medical care of the insured. But their main concern must inevitably be the protection of the funds of the Approved Societies and it is not wholly convincing—at any rate to the doctors—that this should give them the right to control, by a majority representation, the activities of the doctors.

The functions and duties of the insurance committee are defined in the Medical Benefit Regulations which are amended from time to time, and these regulations have been the subject of close consultation with the representatives of the medical profession; so that it would rather appear that the control of the societies in virtue of their majority representation on the committees does not amount to very much in practice. The most important sub-committee of the insurance committee in so far as questions of discipline are concerned is the Medical Service Sub-Committee. Here there is equal representation of the insured persons and the medical profession with an independent chairman.

Complaints against panel doctors.

It will be appreciated that the functions of the Medical Service Sub-committee bear a most important relation to the insurance medical service in each area. Complaints against panel doctors may be made by insured persons, or persons authorised to act on their behalf, or, where irregularities in certification are in question, by Approved Societies. Cases may also be referred by the Insurance Committee to the Medical Service Sub-committee for investigation, but it is not within the function of the sub-committee to make investigations of a general character.

There are reasonable time limits within which complaints must ordinarily be lodged. Hearings are private and, although legal representation is not permitted, the prescribed procedure for the hearings is of a quasi-judicial character. The Medical Service Sub-committee report the result of their investigation, setting out the facts and inferences of fact, and making a recommendation to the Insurance Committee. If a breach of the regulations is established, the doctor may be cautioned or censured by the Insurance Committee and he may be called upon to refund expenses reasonably and necessarily incurred by the insured person, such as payments made to another doctor for his services. A recommendation may also be made to the Minister that a part of the doctor's remuneration should be withheld, and this is quite commonly done, the amounts withheld varying in general from £5 to £20, though smaller or substantially larger sums are occasionally withheld. In the main the cases investigated fall within the following categories:

(*a*) Charging fees to insured persons.

(*b*) Failure to visit patients, or other forms of negligence.

(*c*) Irregularities in certification.

(*d*) Failure to keep records.

Findings of fact by the Medical Service Sub-committee are final. There is a right of appeal to the Minister from the Insurance Committee's recommendation.

My experience, as chairman of the Medical Service Sub-committee for London, leads me to say that those who sit on this tribunal, whether representing insured persons or medical practitioners, are concerned for the good name of the insurance medical service and for the fair treatment of the insured, while always remembering to see that the doctor gets a "square deal".

The Clerk to the London Insurance Committee has provided me with a few extracts from reports by the sub-committee which give a fair sample of the cases which have been investigated from time to time. (These are set out Appendix No. 7). It is hardly necessary to add that in a fair proportion of cases the doctor is found not to have committed any breach of his terms of service.

Removal from the panel.

The disciplinary action taken in the course of the general administration must be sharply distinguished from the more serious question of the removal of a doctor from the panel. It may be noted in this connection that the Minister, although responsible for the spending of public money on the administration of medical benefit, has not the power of selecting the persons by whom the work is to be carried out; every qualified doctor having the right to go on the panel. On the other hand, no doctor can be removed except after the prescribed inquiry. The committee of inquiry consists of a barrister-at-law or a solicitor in actual practice and two medical practitioners. The procedure throughout is judicial, counsel are frequently employed on both sides, and the final decision rests with the Minister after considering the report of the inquiry committee, and taking the opinion of the medical advisory committee, to which reference is made below. The cases where practitioners are so removed are few in number and are usually found to involve grave or persistent failure to provide proper treatment, or personal misconduct of such a character as to bring the service into disrepute.

The doctors' share in the administration.

I have referred in the early part of this chapter to the increasing share in the administration which has been given to the medical profession. The regulations afford evidence that the Minister, in the exercise of his powers under the Acts, is relying more and more on the co-operation of the members of the medical profession themselves, especially where professional questions or professional conduct are at issue. The general interests of the insurance practitioner are looked after by a panel committee in each area, solely representative of the insurance practitioners themselves. This committee must be consulted locally when the terms of service for insurance practitioners are altered. It has representation on the Medical Service Sub-committee which has just been referred to, and is also entrusted with the investigation of alleged extravagant prescribing; and it may act in an advisory capacity to the Insurance Committee on matters (e.g., surgery accommodation) where professional considerations arise. Insurance practitioners act on committees set up by the Minister in connection with the distribution of the available funds for the payment of doctors throughout the country, for special grants in rural areas for mileage, and so on. Further, the Minister has bound himself by regulations to consult a purely medical advisory committee where negligence*, as defined in the regulations, has been alleged against a doctor and the report is before the Minister for consideration.

I believe that the share accorded to the medical profession in the administration is unique. Comparing the English system with all the Continental systems the difference in this respect is very marked and that is doubtless the reason why the doctors here are comparatively satisfied and, in the opinion of many qualified to judge, give a better service.

* Negligence so defined includes :—

Failure to exercise reasonable skill and care in the treatment of a patient.

Failure to visit or treat a patient when necessary.

Failure to order or supply any necessary medicine or appliances for the use of a patient.

Failure to advise the patient as to the steps which should be taken to obtain treatment which is not within the scope of a doctor's terms of service.

Chapter X

Foundations of Medical Benefit

(i) The German System

(ii) The History of Contract Practice

(i) The German System.

Gibbon's book on Medical Benefit in Germany and Denmark, published in 1912, is of great interest, not only because of his very full examination of the question of medical benefit in Germany and Denmark, but because of the conclusions at which he arrives in his various chapters on the questions of a public medical service, to which I make a full reference in a later chapter.

With regard to the medical benefit schemes in Germany and Denmark, Gibbon says:

> "In both Germany and Denmark medical benefit is administered by the societies themselves; there are no intermediate bodies. Terms of service and matters relating to control are arranged directly between the societies and the doctors. It is quite common for the negotiations to be carried out between a federation of societies and an association of doctors; but these act as the agents of the societies and of the doctor.
>
> "The supervisory authorities only intervene in disputes. In Germany, under certain conditions, the authorities may make terms with doctors which the societies within their jurisdiction can be required to observe. But this is only done in extreme cases when there would otherwise be failure on the part of a society to provide adequate medical treatment.
>
> "In Denmark the State has not expressly reserved to itself similar authority, and the intervention of the public authorities is less than in Germany. But the provision of medical benefit is one of the conditions of recognition, and the State has always the power of withdrawing recognition, with consequent loss of subsidy to the society, if satisfactory medical treatment is not provided for members.".

Gibbon sets out the following reasons why in his view it is better for the societies to provide the medical service: —

(*a*) The society can better control the doctors in order to ensure good medical treatment.

(*b*) Adequate medical treatment must include some provision for institutional treatment. This can be much better arranged by a society than by individual members.

(*c*) Supervision is much easier if the society itself arranges for treatment.

(*d*) Malingering is difficult to check. Valetudinarianism still more so. A society can deal with these dangers more effectively if medical services are under its control.

(*e*) Even if the society only gives money benefit, it must still rely largely on the doctor. Money benefit cannot be given, without inviting bankruptcy, except on definite evidence of inability to work. For this purpose medical certificates are necessary, and it is around the giving of such certificates that some of the thorniest problems with regard to the control of the doctors arise.

(*f*) The society can probably arrange more economically for medical treatment, and would be better able to resist exorbitant demands.

(*g*) There would be difficulties in providing benefit if, while the society does not itself provide medical benefit, it nevertheless had to provide money benefit roughly equivalent to the cost of medical treatment.

(*h*) An insurance society, if farsighted, will not content itself simply with the cure of existing ills. It will aim at preventing disease and developing more hygienic habits, and at raising its members to a higher standard of health. (In passing, the present writer may say that in the light of experience of the working of the scheme in this country, this must be regarded as little better than a pious hope).

(*i*) Lastly, there is much more promise of advantage to the community generally when medical treatment is arranged through the society.

One of the needs of the present time, said Gibbon, writing in 1912, is more co-operative organisation..

"As previously stated, a proper balance between the number of doctors required and the number available is much more likely to be secured when arrangements for service are made by the clients, organised in a society, or a federation of societies on the one hand and the doctors organised in their association on the other. More satisfactory terms also can thus be arranged and more efficient service ensured. And such a system holds rich promise of firmer organisation of the medical profession, which, while certainly not without its dangers, should on the whole yield a large margin of gain. The trend of modern conditions is steadily in the direction of such an organisation of both bargaining parties, and it seems highly probable that such a culmination must result if modern tendencies continue to prevail."

The medical profession has in fact become very highly organised by the British Medical Association, although the "bargaining" has from the outset been with the Government and not with the societies.

I do not think that it is necessary to make an extended reference to the question of free choice of doctor which, in Gibbon's book, was said to be one of the bitterest causes of strife between doctors and societies. Generally, the German doctors were strongly for free choice, and the administrators of the societies as strongly against it. Employers were likewise stridently opposed to free choice. It is unnecessary, as I say, to make any examination of this question in detail, because one of the cardinal points laid down by the medical profession when they agreed to work under the insurance scheme in this country was that there should be free choice of doctor; and this is embodied in the scheme as an integral part of the insurance medical service.

These references to the German system and to the problems arising under it are mainly of interest as showing what difficulties had to be avoided in this country, and it is unquestionable that by the devices which were made in 1911-12, such as the creation of local insurance committees, much of the strife and bitterness which spoilt the scheme in Germany did not arise. In fact, at the outset, the German scheme as it existed in 1912 was a valuable guide as to what to avoid rather than what to adopt, and the same might largely be said of our own history of contract practice to which I now make reference.

(ii) The History of Contract Practice.

The earliest complete investigation of the conditions of club practice is contained in a book *The Battle of the Clubs*, published by *The Lancet* in or about 1896. I make the following extract from the Editor's "introduction" to the special commissioner's reports:—

"We venture to think that there are a few morals which may be drawn from this many-sided review of the question:—

"(1) The first and most important is that local combination properly worked will win the day for the practitioner. The medical men, in each neighbourhood where the club system has permeated the routine of practice, should meet and arrange upon their course after due consideration of the situation from every side.

"(2) It is not necessarily disgraceful to be medical officer to a medical aid association, and those who speak and write as if it were take an impractical view.

"(3) These associations are not necessary to the poor, and the philanthropist who asserts that without them those unable to pay large fees to medical men could not obtain medical assistance discourses ignorantly. Many medical men all over the country have clubs of their own where the genuine poor, in return for annual payments suited to their narrow means, are better attended than they are in the big institutions conducted by laymen.

"(4) Nor are these institutions necessary or even useful to the commencing practitioner, as their promoters would have us believe. Such talk is misleading. The regular but paltry pay is only acceptable because no better, under existing conditions, can be obtained. If in a whole neighbourhood the profession stood out against the club system, having first clearly ascertained that abuses were rife under it, the sense of the community would be with the medical men. They would obtain the practice direct instead of through lay committees. And if here and there a bad debt of a few shillings were made owing to the absence of machinery for collecting coppers, many persons well able to afford to pay properly for medical attendance would remunerate the medical man over and over again for his small losses."

The report of the investigation into the economic conditions of contract medical practice made by the British Medical Association in 1905 is a considerable document, from which it is only possible to make a few extracts. The term "contract medical practice" is defined and a very interesting description is given of the various types of organisation with which there had been negotiations from time to time by members of local branches of the British Medical Association, or independently by local practitioners. These were works clubs, provident dispensaries, medical aid societies, the general body of friendly societies in so far as they provided medical benefit, and friendly societies' institutes. Extracts from the report giving descriptions of these various organisations follow:—

Meaning of the term "Contract Medical Practice".

In its widest interpretation the term "contract medical practice" may be held to include any kind of arrangement by which medical practitioners contract with individuals or bodies of the public to render professional services upon conditions, as to remuneration and otherwise, specified in the contract. As thus defined, however, the term would in strictness include the contracts for attendance at fixed annual rates which are entered into by some medical practitioners as a matter of purely private arrangement with individual patients. It would also include the contracts under which medical practitioners are employed by the State, or by municipal and other public authorities, as in the Poor-law Medical Service, and other services of a like character.

Works Clubs.

In these clubs a number of persons engaged in the same employment, taking advantage of a special provision of the Truck

Act, sanction a deduction from their wages for the purpose of providing medical attendance and medicine for themselves alone or for themselves and their families. In some instances the employer himself nominates a "works" doctor; in others each workman is free to nominate any medical practitioner in the district as the person to whom the "stoppage" is to be paid, and no other organization exists beyond the arrangement with the employer to give effect to this agreement; such arrangements closely resemble private clubs in constitution, the medical attendant being actually, if not legally, in direct relation with his patients, without interference from any organized non-medical body.

In other cases mass meetings are held for the election of doctors, and, as the next step in organization, a committee is appointed to watch the interests of the workmen and investigate complaints, but without administrative powers. Arrangements are made for the committee to receive the contributions of the men through the employers, and to disburse the same, paying in some instances for drugs and dispensing, and handing the balance to the medical practitioner or medical practitioners employed. In the fullest development of this system, medical practitioners have been appointed at fixed salaries, their house-rent, rates, and taxes being paid and other allowances made, central dispensaries conducted and hospitals built and managed. In some instances such committees have offered to provide medical attendance and benefits of an allied nature for members of the outside public.

It will be seen that throughout the evolution of such a system it remains governed by the primary fact that the funds by which it is maintained are derived from deductions made from wages for a purpose clearly defined by law, namely, for the provision of medical attendance and medicine for those persons from whose wages the deductions are made, and their dependants. This governing fact differentiates such an organization fundamentally, on the one hand, from Friendly and similar benefit societies in which the provision of medical attendance is only one among many benefits offered, and not even an essential object of the organization, and, on the other hand, from a Provident Dispensary or Medical Aid Society in which the party entering into the contract, as representing the public, is partially or entirely distinct from and independent of the beneficiaries.

Provident Dispensaries.

In these, as in the works clubs, the provision of medical aid is a fundamental and not a subsidiary object, and the beneficiaries have usually some share in the government of the service.

Provident Dispensaries appear to have been established originally as public charities having the object of providing medical attendance for those members of the community who, while not qualified or desiring to receive medical relief under the Poor Law, are believed, nevertheless, to be unable to pay the full cost of the medical attendance which they require. In accordance with this charitable, or partly charitable, origin, representatives of the general public, other than the beneficiaries, usually form a considerable proportion of the governing body. As regards the medical parties to the contract, there are usually several, and in some instances it is open to practically every medical practitioner in the district for which the Dispensary provides to act upon the staff.

Medical Aid Societies.

Medical Aid Societies are bodies formed essentially for the provision of medical attendance, but have not the partly charitable character of Provident Dispensaries, and have as a rule no provision for the representation of the beneficiaries in the government of the society. Many of them are in fact merely bodies trading in medical attendance, either for the purpose of direct profit, or more commonly with the ulterior object of attracting custom for other purposes to the bodies by which their formation is promoted. Thus many Medical Aid Societies have been formed by and closely allied in their working with industrial insurance companies, and the medical aid has been a bait to attract insurers. The management is in the absolute control of the non-medical organizers, and the relation to the profession is correspondingly unsatisfactory.

Medical Aid Societies usually employ only one or two practitioners in each district.

Friendly Societies.

Though the provision of medical aid is not the primary, or even necessary object of friendly and other sick benefit societies.

nevertheless they compose the most widely distributed and perhaps the most numerous group of organizations connected with contract medical practice. The objects of Friendly Societies are, primarily, the insurance of working men, earning weekly wages, against certain misfortunes by which, without such insurance, they may be completely crippled. Friendly Societies, are in fact, mutual assurance societies, in which the system of providing medical attendance has grown up as a natural development of the objects for which they were originally formed.

With them are conveniently considered certain Trades' Unions which provide medical aid as a collateral benefit.

As regards administration, all Friendly Societies are essentially self-governing, but certain differences in the machinery through which the control is exercised affect the relation of these societies to their medical officers. Where there is a national organization the general rules of the Order may restrict the freedom of the local bodies in contracting with their medical officers.

Friendly Societies' Institutes.

In many towns the Friendly Societies have combined for the provision of medical aid, and appoint committees of delegates, to whom the entire organization and management of this part of their work is entrusted. Such committees usually organize central dispensaries and appoint medical officers at fixed salaries, who are required to devote their whole time to the duties of the service.

It is almost impossible to give any clear average of the fees which obtained under the various types of contract practice. Tables given in the appendix to the report exhibit the wide differences which prevail. There are, for example, a few clubs in which the value of the medical officers' services, the supply of medicine included, are assessed at so low a figure as 1/6 per annum; on the other hand what are described as a few highly-favoured practitioners receive as much as 8/8 or even 10/- per annum for attendance on adult males only. The general impression from an examination of the figures is that a good high average rate throughout the whole country was somewhat between 4/- and

5/-; there are very few cases of a rate in force higher than 5/-. (Incidentally, it is to be observed that these low rates which were then in force encouraged the Government to think that the doctors would be ready to come into the scheme of National Health Insurance at what was considered a generous rate of 6/- per annum including drugs.)

The general conclusions arrived at by the investigators included a statement that there was a tendency under the various systems of contract practice to admit persons who were well able to pay the ordinary fees for medical attendance and that this violated the fundamental understanding upon which the medical profession entered into such contracts. It was also suggested that the cause of these evils was the advantage which non-medical organizations were able to take of the competition between individual medical practitioners. The recommendations in substance were that the conditions upon which the medical practitioners in any district undertook contract practice should be prescribed by arrangement amongst themselves, that the general control should be in the hands of some organized local body representative of the profession, and that the medical practitioners of each district should collectively and individually enter into agreements providing, amongst other matters, for rate of remuneration, definition of services to be rendered and tenure of office.

There is no doubt that the conclusions and recommendations embodied in the report of this investigation were of great service to the medical profession, and formed the basis upon which they united in opposition to the terms offered to them under the National Insurance Bill. The action taken by the medical profession in 1911 can be traced in large measure to the recommendations as to organization and definition of terms of service which were set out in that report.

Chapter XI

The Practitioners' Remuneration

Having regard to the information available to the Government as to the rates of pay prevailing in contract practice, Mr. Lloyd George thought at the outset that he would be able to get a really first rate medical service at a rate of 6/- a head including drugs. After a long and wearisome struggle the Exchequer had to supplement insurance funds to the extent of another 2/6, and to this was added the sum of 6d. already available in the calculations as part of the cost of "sanatorium benefit". (This benefit, it will be remembered, did not remain under the insurance scheme for very long.) This made a total of 9/- including drugs.

A short historical note on the capitation fee is set out in Appendix 8, and it may be added that as the result of arbitration in 1937, the capitation fee was fixed at 9/- *excluding drugs*—differing therefore from the 9/- including drugs, which was in force when the Act came into operation. The payment of 9/- was extended to the new class of insured (employed) persons under 16 years of age brought in by the Insurance Act of 1938, although it had been contemplated by the Government that a much smaller capitation fee would have been payable for these young people.

In the course of a review of the financial position which the medical practitioners prepared in support of their case for an increase in the capitation fee put forward in 1923, the doctors' representatives said:—

"It is, or should be, axiomatic that a National Health Insurance Scheme involves the employment of the services of doctors and that those doctors must be properly paid. The amount of their remuneration should be determined on the merits of the case; having been so determined, it should be paid out of the National Health Insurance Fund. It is not conceived that it is within the province of the doctors' representatives to show whether that Fund can stand the burden of this and the other charges properly falling on the Fund; but it does appear to them that the doctors should not be placed in the position of residuary legatees of the Fund after all other charges have been met. It is therefore an essential part of their case that they should not have to look to the Exchequer for the supplementation of the normal Health Insurance Funds for any part of their remuneration; or of appearing to involve demands on funds belonging, whether as of right or of reasonable expectation, to Approved Societies or others."

Amongst the conclusions which were arrived at in that memorandum, it was contended:—

That the amount of the remuneration of the insurance practitioner, having been determined on its merits, must take its place as a charge against the National Health Insurance Fund with all other normal and necessary charges against that Fund.

That there is every indication that the National Health Insurance Fund is in a position of great strength to bear all such charges. (The Government Actuary, writing in March 1922, on the results of the Valuation of Approved Societies as at the end of 1918, had said that "no student of social conditions can fail to be impressed by the financial strength of the system of National Health Insurance",) and

That the favourable results exceeded any reasonable expectations which the societies could have entertained. The question of using these profits to any further extent to pay any part of the cost of Medical Benefit did not arise. But they were such as to enable the societies to face the future with confidence.

In appendix No. 9 a full statement is made with regard to the sums available for medical benefit, and it will be seen that since the year 1927 the cost of medical benefit is directed by statute to be met out of the National Health Insurance Fund, and that a sum of 13/- per annum is earmarked by statute to provide for payments to the doctors and to the chemists and for the expenses of administration.

Although there is provision in the regulations for doctors to be paid under various systems, they have elected everywhere to be paid at a capitation fee for each person, well and ill, on their lists. The dispensing of medicines, except in rural districts, and in certain defined circumstances, is entirely in the hands of the chemists. The capitation fee is supplemented in rural districts by a special payment to doctors for mileage.

The central pool, out of which the doctors are paid, is based on a yearly estimate of the whole insured population made by the Government Actuary. This fund is distributed between the insurance committee areas, and the area pool is distributed amongst the doctors according to the numbers of persons on their respective lists at the beginning of each quarter.

Chapter XII

The Machinery

(a) Certification.

The insurance medical certificate is given on a prescribed form and is a declaration by the doctor that he has examined the patient and that he, or she, is, in that doctor's opinion, incapable of work. The certificates are given in most cases at weekly intervals so long as is necessary, and a " declaring-off " certificate is required when the patient is fit to resume work.

The first concern of the doctor must, of course, be to see that no insured person is at work when he is not fit, but he has also to realise that every certificate which he gives is in substance a cheque entitling the insured person to payment out of insurance funds, and that he must, therefore, give his certificate fairly and conscientiously. The increasing demands made upon National Health Insurance sickness funds in recent years have been the subject of much concern to the authorities. The appointment of Regional Medical Officers of the Ministry as referees on the subject of incapacity for work—their principal but not their only function—has led to an enormous number of claims coming under review, and, in quite a large proportion of the cases sent to these referees, the patient who has been certified by his panel doctor to be incapable of work has either not presented himself for examination by the referee or on examination has been found not to be incapable of work. (In fairness it must be recognised that some days elapse between the case being certified and the date for the referee's examination). This machinery resulted in a substantial check on loose certification but was found to be insufficient.

A procedure was, therefore, introduced by regulation which was analogous to that which had already been in force for some years with regard to excessive prescribing. The procedure is as follows:

> There is first an investigation of the facts affecting individual practitioners; this is carried out generally by the regional medical staff, and would normally arise out of the observation

by the regional medical officer of a large number of references on incapacity (made by approved societies) in the case of the the same practitioner. Following this investigation, those cases which appear to call for further action are referred to the panel committee. It is the duty of the panel committee to send to the practitioner a statement of those matters in respect of which the Department has indicated that explanation is required and to give the practitioner an opportunity of submitting a statement in writing, or of being heard by the panel committee. There is a right of appeal to the Minister against the panel committee's findings and recommendation.

Some of the explanations given to regional medical officers by a number of practitioners have been thought worthy of inclusion in the official memorandum issued in 1931, 329/I.C.,—to which extensive reference has already been made in the chapter on the control of sickness benefit claims—drawing attention to a marked and continuous rise in sickness benefit claims. The statements made by practitioners included the following:—

That they found themselves unable to certify strictly in accordance with their medical judgment for fear of losing patients.

That when their patients complained of illness and inability to work they did not feel justified, even in the absence of any signs of disease, in refusing certificates.

That, although they might believe a patient to have recovered and become able to resume work, they preferred to leave the duty of saying so to the examining officer of the Department.

That, although a patient might legitimately be considered to be not incapable of work, the doctor knew how difficult it would be for that patient to find work under the prevailing conditions of employment, and he allowed himself to be influenced by compassionate considerations.

In the memorandum it is pointed out that the standard, by which certain practitioners are judged to have failed to exercise proper care in the issue of certificates, is that which is afforded by comparison of their work with that of their colleagues.

I have dealt at some length, in the chapter on the control of sickness benefit claims, see page 115, with the disturbing character of the results of the references to the regional medical staff of certificates of incapacity issued by insurance practitioners. I may add here that from the reports of the Department for the year 1937, it appears that out of a total of 543,000 cases referred to the Regional Medical Staff, 212,000 resulted in the insurance practitioner's certificate being confirmed, and the remaining 331,000 cases are those of insured persons who either received a "declaring-off" certificate before the date fixed for the examination, or did not attend the examination, or on attendance were found not to be incapable of work. In these figures it is noteworthy that there is a considerable preponderance in the number of women as compared with men.

It is an interesting reflection that when the Regional Medical Staff was first appointed, stress was laid on the advice and help which they would give to insurance practitioners just as much as on their functions of inspection and control of sickness benefit claims; and it was hoped that insurance practitioners would make full use of the services of these regional officers. Unfortunately this has not proved to be the case. The number of "consultation" references made by insurance practitioners to the Regional Medical Staff in 1937 was 377 only, and of these no less than 316 cases were referred by doctors in Scotland, and the total number of cases in which practitioners themselves sought the opinion of the Regional Medical Officer on the question of incapacity was 3,100 only as compared with over half a million cases referred by the approved societies.

As to the cases referred by the Approved Societies, it can only be said that the proportion of the cases in which patients declared off the funds is still alarmingly high, and that, although the new arrangements for the review of individual practitioners' certification have been in force for four or five years, and the number of cases investigated by the regional medical staff is doubtless considerable, there is no published record of this or of any action following the regional medical officers' investigation which has been taken by the panel committees in any instance. The question, therefore, of the continuance of the claims for sickness and disablement benefit which continue to be largely in excess of expectation is a matter which is still giving the authorities a good deal of anxiety. For example, in March 1938 the Department wrote to the Insurance Acts Committee of the British Medical Association stating that the Minister was deeply concerned at the extent to which incapacitating illness of long duration continued among the insured population, with all that is entailed by way of deterioration in health and loss of earnings, and that he would like to have more precise information on the problem than is at present available; and inviting the co-operation of the Insurance Acts Committee in the investigation which was proposed.

(*b*) *Prescribing.*

One of the fundamental principles in the National Health Insurance Scheme is that prescribing and dispensing are required to be separated, the dispensing being done by pharmacists who have entered into agreements and placed their name on the panel of pharmacists. There are three exceptions. The practitioner himself is required to supply, and not merely to prescribe, (*a*) those drugs and appliances which are necessarily or ordinarily administered by a practitioner in person, (*b*) all drugs and appliances in rural districts where pharmacists are not available, and (*c*) in all districts, drugs, etc., which are required for immediate use when the pharmacists' shops are closed, or in an emergency.

It is inevitable in a national system affecting the whole working population that some checks on extravagant prescribing should be imposed. The uninformed criticism which is directed to the provisions under the scheme in this respect was answered by the Chairman of the Insurance Acts Committee of the British Medical Association in a published letter of the 1st December 1930. After referring to a recent letter in the public press as "an entirely misleading and erroneous statement, based on a case of proved extravagance in prescribing," he says "A panel doctor can, and mostly does, treat his panel patients in the same way as his private patients, and he may, and frequently does, order for them the most expensive remedies known to medicine, the only limit placed upon him being that, if challenged, he can satisfy, not the officers of the Ministry, but his own colleagues, that what he has ordered was reasonably necessary for the treatment of his patients." The machinery under the regulations does provide, as stated in that letter, for the control of extravagance in prescribing by the practitioner's own colleagues. The drugs, etc., must be those which are "requisite for the treatment of the patient", and the cost must not be in excess "of what is reasonably necessary for adequate treatment," but no limits are imposed anywhere as to the cost of any drug which may be supplied or as to the average cost of the drugs supplied free of charge to insured persons, and official rulings have placed beyond doubt that the practitioner himself must be the judge in the first instance of what is necessary for his patients; he is in fact expected to exercise the same discretion as when providing for his private patients from his own stock of medicines. The terms of the Act itself require that insured persons shall have "proper and sufficient" medicines.

With regard to the cost of prescribing, there is no need, as it has been done so often, to present volumes of figures or to quote extensive extracts from the reports, in which admonitions are repeated as to the excessive cost of prescribing on the part of many insurance practitioners, and to the tendency in some quarters to prescribe extravagant proprietary medicines. One fact which emerges from the published reports is that in England and Wales the yearly cost of prescribing per head of the insured population is approximately 3/-, and in Scotland 2/-. This disturbing fact calls for the close attention of all who are engaged in insurance practice. With an estimated population in England and Wales of 15,000,000 insured persons, the excess in the cost of prescribing as compared with Scotland represents an additional annual charge of no less than £750,000. The excess is due to differences in methods of prescribing in the two countries and should not be beyond the competence of representatives of the medical profession to reduce or even to eliminate.

A memorandum from the Ministry of Health issued in December, 1936, deals with various aspects of the problem of excessive prescribing, and an extract is given hereunder. The question also received considerable attention from the Scottish Department of Health, notwithstanding the fact that the costs in Scotland compared so very favourably with those in England.

Extract from Memorandum from Ministry of Health (December 1936) on the Cost of Prescribing.

1. The continuous increase in the cost of prescribing for insured persons is causing concern to all engaged in the adminis-

tration of medical benefit, and it is noted that public expression has been given by various bodies and persons to the suggestion that the efforts of the Department to control excessive prescribing should be supplemented by the help of other bodies. In particular, the chairman of the Insurance Acts Committee has publicly claimed that the profession itself, if given an opportunity, can help materially. It is in view of these expressions of opinion that the Department asks for the co-operation of the Insurance Acts Committee and submits the following notes for its consideration.

2. The problem of the investigation of the rising costs of prescribing presents itself in two aspects: (*a*) the differences observed between the prescribing costs of individual practitioners within an area, and (*b*) the wide differences between the average prescribing costs in different areas of the country.

3. Cases of apparently excessive cost arising under the first head lend themselves to treatment under Article 42 of the Medical Benefit Consolidated Regulations, 1928, which contemplates that panel committees will address their minds in a judicial manner to the evidence submitted to them with a view to deciding what excessive cost (if any) has been imposed on medical benefit funds, having regard to such standard of comparison as is available to the committees—which is normally the average cost in their area.

4. There remains the difficult problem of the wide variations between areas. It is common ground that the cost of prescribing must be expected to vary with the type of area, and that the costs in industrial areas will be in excess of those in rural areas by reason, mainly, of the incidence of morbidity, mass psychology, and accessibility to medical advice. There are, however, marked differences as between areas which are similar in their industrial characteristics.

8. The number of prescriptions issued obviously depends on the two factors of (*a*) the number of insured persons applying for treatment, and (b) the number of prescriptions given to each person treated. The first factor is only to a limited extent within the practitioner's control; the second is largely within his discretion. Turning to the marked differences between the areas, it is clear that if this could be shown to be due solely to the proportion of insured persons seeking treatment there would be no case for inquiry so far as the cost of prescribing is concerned.

The evidence, however, does not suggest this, but rather the contrary. Certain areas reasonably comparable as regards industrial conditions, but differing widely as regards prescribing costs, have been selected, and the medical records of practitioners who are known to keep good records have been examined in each area. The results are shown in the following table.*

9. The evidence from this table seems to show that there are factors *under the control of the practitioners* which account for some of the variations in prescribing costs in different areas of the country. It is not apparent why Rochdale with 60 per cent. of insured persons treated annually should show 4.8 prescriptions per insured person, while Salford with approximately the same proportion treated, requires seven prescriptions. Similar discrepancies reveal themselves between Blackburn and Bolton, Leeds and Wakefield, Birmingham and Wolverhampton.

10. These are the problems upon which it is hoped the Insurance Acts Committee, in the light of experience and after making such inquiries as they may think expedient, may be in a position to throw some light, with a view to suggesting in particular any measures which they may consider practicable for reducing the costs in areas with abnormally high averages.

(*c*) *Records of illness.*

The keeping of records is one of the conditions of insurance practice which most doctors frankly dislike. The obligation, however, is not a very exacting one, and is actually welcomed by those practitioners—though they are only too few—who realise the value of method and order in their practice. The obligation involves keeping in alphabetical order the cards for each patient. These cards are supplied to the doctor with the particulars in regard to the insured person already written up, and he is expected as a matter of routine to put a tick in one or more of the three columns, attendance, visit, and certificate, on each occasion when he sees a patient. He is also—and this is the principal purpose of the record—expected to keep a short clinical note, but only where in his judgment it is likely to be of service to himself or another doctor for reference on future occasions. The making of the routine entries (the ticks) on the card, if they are made at the time of seeing the patient, should ensure that the doctor has

* Not reproduced here.

in front of him any past clinical notes. As the card is a continuous record of the patient's medical history, intended to last for the whole of his life, being passed on from doctor to doctor it is obvious that in later illnesses these cards should, if properly kept, be a valuable source of information to the doctor. (The record on the card is confidential). The record of attendances, visits and certificates—again if properly kept—should also be of much value for administrative and statistical purposes.

With regard to the value of these records for statistical purposes, the only occasion so far as I am aware on which they have been used for the purposes of an enquiry was with regard to the incidence of rheumatic diseases.

In 1922 the Ministry of Health closely investigated a "sample" of 90,000 persons coming within the purview of the National Health Insurance Act. The insured population at that date numbered about 13,500,000; so the sample represented less than 7 per cent. The survey was over a period of one year only; and it was faced with the familiar difficulty of the lack of a perfected classification in this group of diseases. Yet the survey was able to arrive at a statistical result which can be accepted as approximating to correctness, especially as it coincides with the results of somewhat similar investigations in other countries. The conclusions were that rheumatic disease was probably responsible for 16 per cent. of the total of industrial morbidity in England and Wales, and that during the course of a year about 372,600 insured persons sought medical advice because of some form of rheumatic disease. The highest incidence was among metal workers, transport workers, agricultural workers, mine workers, building workers, and clerical workers, in that order.

It is hardly to be doubted that with the continuous attention which the regional medical staff are giving to the way in which insurance practitioners keep their records there must be a considerable improvement in the keeping of these records in recent years. At the same time there is, in well-advised quarters, a definite opinion that the only results of real value to be obtained in this connection would be secured by having records thoroughly kept by a selected number of insurance practitioners, who would have to be, presumably, specially remunerated for this work, rather than records kept as a matter of routine by every insurance practitioner, in most cases without enthusiasm.

Chapter XIII

A short note on Maternity Benefit

Maternity Benefit is a cash payment of forty shillings on the confinement of an insured woman or of the wife of an insured man. Medical treatment in respect of a confinement forms no part of the treatment which an insured doctor is required to give under his contract.

It is obvious that the question of making better provision for maternity is one related to the maternity and child welfare work* of the local authorities. In the meantime I may note the following extracts from the report of the Royal Commission.

> (P. 50). "No survey of the health services under the Insurance Act would be complete if it omitted to take account of maternity benefit. It is true that this is a cash benefit administered directly by the Approved Societies, and that it differs from the additional treatment benefits in that there is no control of the application of the money given. Yet the money does in large part go to pay for the services of the doctor and midwife and the underlying purpose of the benefit is to promote the health of mother and child at the critical period of pregnancy and childbirth. Having regard to the great importance of skilled advice and treatment at that time, we feel confident that any development of this benefit will be in the direction of an increase of the service element provided under appropriate conditions of control.

* The great improvement effected in maternity and child welfare provision dates from Mr. Herbert (now Lord) Samuel's presidency of the Local Government Board. (1914).

The number of maternity and child welfare centres increased from a few hundreds in 1912 to 2,172 in 1922, and 6,487 in 1942.

The death rate among infants under a year of age has fallen as follows :—

1912	95 per thousand
1922	77 per thousand
1942	49 per thousand

The deaths of women attributed to pregnancy and child-bearing have been—

1912	3,629,
1922	3,105
1942	1,669

(The figures are given in Viscount Samuel's Memoirs—Cresset Press, 1945).

"The B.M.A. recommend that in addition to a cash payment there should be suitable ante-natal examination and supervision, attendance at confinement and during the puerperal period by a midwife or doctor as the case requires, consultant and specialist services available for difficult cases, and provision for institutional treatment where necsessary."

The Society of Medical Officers of Health who, as representing the medical advisers of the bodies responsible for the work of the Maternity and Child Welfare Centres, speak with special authority in this matter, say that "the maternity and child welfare schemes have involved local authorities in large expenditure frequently greatly exceeding the total amount of maternity benefit paid in their district." They point out that "These schemes are of the same essential nature as maternity benefit and the only practical method by which this latter benefit can be administered in the interests of the mother and child is by requiring local authorities to administer it through their statutory Maternity and Child Welfare Committees." After reciting the need for the same elements of medical attention as those recommended by the British Medical Association they go on to say that "maternity benefit even in money value should vary according to the necessity of the mother and the medical character of the case." They conclude with the following recommendations:—

"Maternity benefit, whether in its present, or in an extended form, should cease to be administered by Approved Societies and be administered both in money and kind by local authorities; which, in their turn, should be made definitely responsible for providing medical attention. The attendance upon maternity cases should not be an obligation upon a panel practitioner.

Maternity benefit should provide for all necessary medical attendance in pregnancy and maternity, and medical benefit should be understood to be exclusive of such medical attendance."

CHAPTER XIV

THE INSURANCE MEDICAL SERVICE—SOME CONCLUSIONS AND CRITICISMS

Although the Royal Commission, so far as the machinery of the Insurance Medical Service is concerned, recommended that insurance committees should be abolished and their powers transferred to the local authorities, the Commission had no criticism to offer with regard to the character of the service given by the general body of insurance practitioners. They find, as indeed they were bound to find, that the service itself was seriously incomplete. It is possible to criticize the service from this point of view— this being a matter in which the doctors have no control— while recognising that within the scope of the existing contract the doctors are giving as reasonably good service as could fairly be expected. I append one or two extracts from the Royal Commission's report. I have already made an extended reference to what the late Sir Henry Brackenbury had to say on the subject in his book "Patient and Doctor". (See Ch. 9).

(R.C. p. 36). "We turn now to a new subject on which there has been, and may still be, a certain amount of public misgiving. We refer to the suggestion frequently made in the early days of the scheme and still heard occasionally, that doctors and chemists deliberately give to insured persons a service inferior to that given to their private patients. We are glad to say that, except for some rather contradictory evidence given by witnesses from the National Conference of Friendly Societies, we have found no support for this allegation. On the contrary, there has been a great body of evidence not only from the interested parties—the doctors and chemists—but from societies and representative bodies showing that no such distinction is made.

It is, perhaps, proper to observe that in a service comprising 15,000 doctors it is impossible to postulate that all will, at all times and in all circumstances, maintain a superlative standard of efficiency and care. The medical profession, like every other craft and calling, can claim no immunity from the intrusion of undesirable and unworthy elements. Nor does this imply any disrespect towards an honourable profession; it is merely an acknowledgment of their common humanity. Isolated cases of negligence and carelessness, therefore, prove nothing; such occur in private practice also. Even if it were established statistically that there were proportionately more causes of complaint in insurance practice than in private practice, this, again, would in itself prove nothing. The causes of complaint might be due to the industrial or social peculiarities of certain areas or to the idiosyncrasies of certain doctors, and these might manifest themselves irrespective of the arrangements under which the doctor was giving his service. As against the rather vague suggestions that have been made, it is only right to refer to one other consideration put in evidence before us, namely, that there is a growing tendency among practitioners to be more scrupulous to avoid giving offence in the case of insurance patients than in the case of private patients, since the former are, in a sense, protected by the machinery under the Act for the investigation of complaints."

The Acceptance of the Act by the Profession.

It may be that long and close association with the service actually results in my critical faculties becoming dulled or even inoperative. So far, however, as my judgment goes, the present system has appeared to meet all the reasonable requirements of the medical profession. The large share in administration which, as we have seen, the doctors enjoy, the complete freedom from interference where the exercise of professional judgment is involved, the right of the patient to choose his own doctor, and that of the doctor within wide limits to reject patients that he does not want, the simple and straightforward character of the requirements in regard to the certification and records—all combine to make the service as satisfactory to those engaged in it as can be expected, when proper allowance for human nature is made. This has been frankly placed on record on many occasions by the Insurance Acts Committee of the British Medical Association, though, of course, from time to time they reserve for continued criticism many matters of detail. It seems equally true that criticism of the service from those medical men not engaged in it is now confined to very few and occasional critics whose observations, often ill-informed and twisted out of any real resemblance to the facts as they are, make it difficult to treat them seriously.

I want to stress the fact that the doctor's first concern is the welfare of his patient, and that an insurance contribution is merely one method of paying the doctor for his services. Since the Act came into operation there has arisen a new generation of medical men who regard the insurance system and this method of payment for their services as a definite and permanent part of our social system, and it is difficult to suppose nowadays that a medical man is likely to give one kind of service to a patient for whom he is paid an insurance premium, and another kind of service to a patient who happens to pay a fee for each attendance. It might be expected that human nature is such that a doctor would give better service where he is paid a fee for each service, but in the long run, in a properly organised medical service, there should be no real distinction between the kind of service that the doctor gives where he is paid by an insurance premium, and that where he is paid by fees. The medical profession have accepted service under a code of regulations, dealing with a great range of matters, which mean nothing more than this, that if a medical man goes about his job as he would in private practice, and gives the same reasonable amount of care and attention to his patient, he need have no fear that he is likely to be infringing any of the regulations. All that he needs to do is to carry out his work efficiently, according to the dictates of his own conscience and the traditions of the profession, and it will be found that, except in regard to certain matters with which he must make himself acquainted, such as his responsibility for giving certificates of incapacity, keeping records, and writing prescriptions, he will not run any risk of breaking the law.

Criticism from the Insured and Employers.

The criticism of the service from the insured population and their employers, who watch the working of the panel system with a good deal of interest, is rather on a different footing. It is impossible not to recognize that, even to-day, there is a good deal of dissatisfaction with the service. Only a fraction of it emerges in the shape of formal complaints, and it is probably more apparent in areas where the insurance work forms only a relatively small part of the general practitioner's practice than in those large industrial areas where the panel work is heavy and practically every doctor in the area is engaged in it. With regard to this dissatisfaction there are two possible explanations. The first is that where a doctor is treating for an insurance premium patients for whom he formerly received—often from the employer—fairly substantial fees, he has not yet got over a certain amount of resentment or a feeling that he has not been fairly treated; this observation applies to a steadily diminishing group, as the younger men who have grown up with the capitation system may be expected not to have this feeling. The second is that insured persons or their employers are sometimes unduly exacting and are inclined to require with some impatience that a doctor should do this thing or that, where formerly, when there was no pre-existing contractual relationship, there would be an invitation rather than a request to see a patient and a more ready recognition of the fact that the hard-worked doctor had plenty of other calls on his time. This merely amounts to saying that there are two sides to the question and it will, therefore, entirely fail to satisfy either those persons who say that you can expect no good from a "panel doctor", or those doctors who are very angry with insured persons who are always insisting on their "rights".

I give here a quotation from the P.E.P. report dealing with the case against National Health Insurance, and for a public medical service.

"The case against the insurance system and its extension is based, according to the Committee on the Scottish Health Services, on some of the following arguments:

(1) Medical services, like elementary education, should be free to all members of the community;

(2) To extend the National Health Insurance system to cover the greater part of the population would be merely a wasteful administrative measure, since it would create machinery to exclude a very small number of people;

(3) It is cheaper to levy rates and taxes than to raise contributions;

(4) Contributory insurance should be kept for the expansion of pensions and other benefits, and therefore it is un-

desirable to exhaust the contributory power of the wage-earning classes in providing medical services;

(5) Medical services under a contributory system are given not according to need but according to insurance status, which depends on factors such as employment having no relation to health;

(6) All the health services should be unified under the local and central authorities.

"Perhaps the most fundamental objection to the extension of medical services by extending the system of National Health Insurance is that it might hinder a proper overhauling and integration of all the medical services. This consideration weighed heavily with those who signed the Majority Report of the Royal Commission on National Health Insurance. In taking a very wide view they said: 'In particular we feel sure that the wider the scope of these services (i.e., the health services) the more difficult will it be to retain the insurance principle. The ultimate solution will be, we think, in the direction of divorcing the medical services entirely from the insurance system and reorganising it along with all the other public health activities as a service to be supported from the general public funds'. They reached this conclusion partly as a result of observing that the distinction between the health services which benefited the community, such as the environmental services, and the health services such as the medical service which benefited only the individual, was rapidly breaking down.

"The alternative plans for extending medical provision by creating a comprehensive public medical service differ in their financial details and in their proposed relation to the existing insurance service. The general principle on which they would be based is the creation of a public medical service available to all persons. There would be, as far as possible, free choice of a doctor, and a doctor would be paid from a central fund either on a capitation basis or on any other system acceptable both to the State and to the profession.

"The doctor would, of course, pass persons on to specialist institutions whenever that was necessary, and co-ordination and the elimination of overlapping between the general practitioner service and the institutional service would thus be secured.

"The service would be financed by some combination of State grants, contributions from local rates and recovery of costs from patients treated, which last would inevitably involve some kind of means test. Difficulty would arise in relating any such scheme to the existing National Health Insurance system. One possibility would be to abolish health insurance and compensate the existing contributors by guaranteeing them an appropriate measure of unconditional free benefit. This would secure a really comprehensive medical service. A less drastic alternative would be to keep the existing scheme and to confine the public service to uninsured persons and to insured persons not already covered for the treatment in question. This would evidently give rise to an unfortunate administrative dualism, since health insurance would be preserved and another service would be set up alongside it.

"Even if it were conveniently possible to find the necessary funds for a public medical service from some source other than insurance, is is plain that the prior existence of a great and deeply rooted national health insurance system would be a very serious obstacle. But the surmounting of this obstacle hardly seems worth serious examination because there is an even greater difficulty to be met first.

"The crux of the problem is finance. Extended general practitioner and other medical services are bound to cost more. How and from whom is the additional money to be raised? It seems unlikely that the State and local authorities could afford to shoulder the burden under existing circumstances. For some considerable time to come the service would have to be at least partially financed by the patients' own payments. Thus the argument, that a free State service comparable to the educational service would be provided, breaks down. The state of public finances would not permit it. There is no reason to suppose that payments for services rendered are cheaper to collect than contributions, nor would it be considered equitable to charge directly a person earning £150 per annum the same as a person earning £250 per annum. To meet this difficulty a means test would have to be introduced, and a means test always discourages the use of even an essential service. Further, the charge for medical services would fall on the family at a time of economic strain, particularly if the breadwinner had suffered from illness.

"If these arguments are valid it seems that the least burdensome way of raising the necessary sum would be through a more comprehensive scheme of contributory insurance. In fact the working-class are prepared to pay considerable premiums for medical insurance without any form of means test. Insurance payments are popular but means tests, however mild, have become odious. Hence the extraordinary popularity of the hospitals contributory schemes, with nearly 5¼ million subscribers of between 2d. and 4d. a week. These payments give the subscribers the right to free treatment in voluntary and very often in public hospitals without any inquiries into means by the hospital almoner.

"Very large numbers of people are not covered at all by National Health Insurance, and those who are covered still find themselves left to meet much of their sickness risk both as regards treatment and loss of income. A further extension was brought about by the raising of the limit of remuneration of non-manual workers from £250 to £420 per annum. One extension, to wage-earners aged between 14 and 16, has lately been initiated by the Government in the National Health Insurance (Juvenile Contributors and Young Persons) Bill"—now an Act which came into force in April, 1938.

The Royal Commission appeared to be in no doubt that ultimately the medical service would have to be divorced from the insurance system.

(p. 65): "The ultimate solution will lie, we think, in the direction of divorcing the medical service entirely from the insurance system and recognising it along with all the other public health activities as a service to be supported from the general funds. Consideration would have to be given to the question of the classes of society for whom the service would be available and whether it should be so available on a free basis or with payments by insurance or otherwise. These, however, are problems which need not—perhaps cannot—be solved now, but may be fitly left over for those who, unlike us, will approach at close range to the question of the Public Health Service of the future."

Chapter XV

Progress towards an Organised Medical Service for the Nation.

Before reciting the objections to a public medical service, which are well summarised in Gibbon's book,* I think it desirable to quote a statement which he makes with regard to the fact that the provision of medical benefit through insurance presents formidable problems, but that some of these problems at any rate do not arise wholly from insurance. They are inherent in existing social conditions. Insurance does but focus and intensify them. At the same time, by the very fact of doing so, it affords better opportunities for systematic efforts at solution. What is of essential importance is that the broad principles of action should be well and truly planned, and that the general direction should be judiciously mapped out. That done, however, the mistakes and mishaps that may happen by the way can be effectively remedied by wise ingenuity.

Here is Gibbon's summary of the objections to what he calls a unified public system:—

"(*a*) There is danger that a unified public system would become unified to stolidity. Service might conceivably be fairly efficient for a generation. But there is little doubt that it would tend to become stereotyped. It would become immune to new ideas, and in medicine, as in other spheres, it is the new idea which counts most for progress.

(*b*) It is doubtful whether it would maintain a high standard of efficiency even for one generation. Valetudinarianism, that habit of mind which exaggerates ills and creates others of their own imagination, might become rampant. Malingering would also probably be a grave evil, though less serious than valetudinarianism.

(*c*) The plea for a public service is based largely on what is essentially a primitive view of hygiene. It leans on the notion that the material environment is the most important matter. But

* See Introductory Note to Part 2.

modern research is all in the direction of showing that other factors are much more important—personal hygiene, which depends on character and the subtle make-up of mind, and conditions of heredity. Character and the sub-conscious foundation of good habits are best acquired in active self-government, whether individual or as a member of a society or group.

(*d*) Under a public medical service, the power of the doctor would be very great. Dealing with the intimate concerns of life, it might well become intolerable.

(*e*) The notion that a unified state service would be economical is probably a delusion. There would almost surely be a large increase of work. Much service would almost certainly be only mildly efficient. The general standard of work, in quality as well as quantity, would probably be less in a public service, with its sheltered security, than under a more strenuous system.

(*f*) Lastly, against the ideal of a community in which functions are concentrated under governmental control may be set an ideal in which persons are organised in self-governing groups according to their functions, needs and interests, and all these groups organised in turn into a co-operative whole for the common good."

I think that I should here interpose at once some reference to this question of the government by groups. We have already seen how the idea of government by the insured members themselves in the scheme as a whole disappeared into thin air when the Industrial Assurance Companies and the Collecting Societies came on the scene. The medical profession in this country were quite determined not to work under the control of Approved Societies, and their objection was sustained, so that separate bodies had to be set up in order to administer medical benefit. These were the Insurance Committees, whose abolition was recommended by the Royal Commission in 1926; their powers to be transferred to the local authorities. The fact that no such transfer has been made, and that Insurance Committees are still very much alive, may to some extent be attributed to the fact that, whereas the medical profession would regard themselves, if under the control of Approved Societies, as being chastised by whips, they would look upon the control of the local authorities, as they at present exist, as chastisement by scorpions.

For those who entertain the view that expenditure on health services is a substantial contribution to national economy, the observations of Sir Andrew Duncan and Professor Alexander Gray in their statement of reservations to the Report of the Royal Commission, will repay careful study—they say (p. 294):

> "Expenditure on social services is not infrequently supported by reference to the economies which will elsewhere result; it is difficult, viewing the matter retrospectively, to find instances where such hopes have been adequately realised. As our health services are at present organised, we see little to support the view that expenditure on health now would lead to a diminution on health in the future. On the contrary, there are grounds for believing that expenditure on health, unless primarily directed to the removal of the causes of ill-health, may tend to occasion a further increase in such expenditure. These observations are not to be taken as implying that there is not a strong case for expenditure on health services, or even that a case might not be made out for regarding such expenditure as so urgent as to constitute the first call on the country's resources. With that particular question we are not at the moment concerned . We merely desire to point out that the case for expenditure on health is not in fact furthered by what, we are convinced, is the fallacious suggestion that expenditure on health may directly help to rehabilitate the finances of the the country."

I make here a further extract from Sir Henry Brackenbury's book: —

> "It is not possible at present to forecast with any great degree of accuracy the exact character of the future organization of medical services in the interest of the general community. It is certain that such organization will continue to develop. The State will not cease to concern itself either with the public health, or with the health of the individual citizen, in so far as these two spheres can be distinguished from one another. More and more will the preventive and the perfective or constructive aspects of medicine be insisted upon, and increasingly will the State make it its business to see that every citizen has full

opportunity of receiving adequate and suitable medical advice and treatment. The extent and direction to which anything of this sort will be done in the immediate future depend upon financial exigencies and social views. At the moment it is profitable to examine the requirements and relations of patient and doctor, of the community and the organized medical profession, to discover from the mass of previous experience what are the features of those relations which seem most worth preserving, and to lay down certain general principles which should guide, on the one hand, the patient seeking and using a doctor, and, on the other hand, the State in organizing and using the services of the medical profession as a whole for the purposes of the public health and welfare.

"With the patient as a unit in a social system there are many others besides the doctor who may have very great, even paramount, responsibility. The educational influence of the teacher, the spiritual influence of the clergyman or minister, the psychological influence of both these and of others, are instruments of the greatest importance; and in the social sphere there are numbers of persons—sometimes too many, almost a multitude—who may have to do with the patient and may greatly affect the situation. The doctor, as well as the patient, has to take all these into account, and they have to take the doctor into account: so that he becomes, in a large number of cases, if not in most, not a solitary worker but one of a team. In these circumstances two things are necessary for the welfare of the patient. One is that the principal responsibility should remain with one person, the leader of the team. The other is that each worker, the doctor as well as all the others, should be skilled at his own business and not encroach upon the field of others."

In this twentieth century, Organisation becomes more and more the watchword in every form of industrial and social life and we are rapidly getting away from the old idea that it was sufficient somehow to muddle through. We shall be compelled by the march of events—and I am sure that the time is not very far distant—to establish organised health services everywhere throughout the land, and to bring them under the ultimate control of a body which is the Ministry of Health, and not also a Ministry of a good many other things. Insurance, I have suggested, will have to find its place under some other departmental control, e.g., that of a Minister of Social Insurance, and the question of the medical service will have to be settled as a major question of health services, and not as a mere piece of the insurance machinery as it is at present. The one vital connecting link between the insurance medical service and the insurance cash benefit is the doctor's certificate of incapacity, and in the opinion of many observers well qualified to judge, the fact that a doctor has to give a certificate of incapacity before a cash payment can be made, and that every medical certificate which he gives is virtually a cheque drawn on the funds of Approved Societies, does not justify bringing the health service itself under the control of the Approved Societies, either directly or indirectly. Certification, as I have said elsewhere, can be arranged between the Insurance authority and the Health authority and most effectively controlled by the latter.

Organisation does not mean bringing the whole medical profession into one regimented service with definite scales of salary, but that, within the scheme of a national organised medical service, it is essential to make adequate provision for linking up the general practitioner with specialists and institutional services and to finance such a scheme on the theory that health is the first consideration and that everyone should contribute to the health service as a whole.

It is a self-evident truth that the health of the people is the concern of the whole community. Without health, all other things—empire, armaments, religion, the happiness of the people —are impossible of attainment.

If that be accepted, we must progress, and progress rapidly, towards an organised medical service for the nation.

The health of the whole body corporate is a national concern, not susceptible of varying standards in different parts of the country and not to be tinkered with by reason of prejudices of the medical profession, or the play of politics. It is true, as it was in the day of Disraeli, that "the first consideration is the health of the people."

CHAPTER XVI

(September 1945)

A COMPLETE NATIONAL HEALTH SERVICE

It is possible now to write that the comprehensive medical service for the community towards which it has been noted that we have been travelling is about to be attained. The Government have announced that they intend to establish a National Health Service, which will provide for *everyone* all the medical advice, treatment, and care that they may require. The necessary legislative provision will be introduced early in the new Parliament.

In the White Paper issued in 1944 it is stated that

> "in considering the form which the new National Health service should take, the Government had the help of informal discussions (in no way binding on those who took part in them) with representatives of the major Local Authorities, the Medical Profession, the Voluntary Hospitals and others. They now put forward definite proposals for discussion in Parliament and in the country, but they do not at this stage put the proposals forward as fixed decisions. Indeed, they have promised that those concerned, professionally or otherwise, shall be fully consulted before final decisions are taken. The Government will welcome constructive criticism and they hope that the next stage—the stage of consultation and public discussion—will enable them to submit quickly to Parliament legislative proposals which will be largely agreed."

The medical profession may fairly claim that for a quarter of a century they have fully explored the ground, and have made a substantial contribution towards the establishment of a comprehensive service. In the report of the council of the British Medical Association drawn up in 1944, in response to the Government's invitation of constructive criticism, it is stated:—

> "The medical profession is in complete agreement with the Government's aim to ensure that every man, woman, and child should be able to obtain all the advice and treatment and care

which they may need in matters of health, and that the country's full resources are brought to bear upon reducing ill-health and promoting good health in all its citizens. The profession, particularly in the last quarter of a century, has again and again pressed upon the Government of the day developments and amplifications of health provision to this end. That pressure has been almost without avail. For example, the Interim Report of the Consultative Council on Medical and Allied Services (the Dawson Report) in 1920 outlined a scheme of primary and secondary health centres; the British Medical Association in 1930 and again in 1938 published its "General Medical Service for the Nation" which recommended the integration and co-ordination of the medical services; and in 1942 the Medical Planning Commission issued a Draft Interim Report which made further proposals for the reorganisation of the medical services. All these documents were submitted to the Government for consideration."

A close examination has been made by the present writer on many occasions of the various documents which have been produced in the course of the B.M.A. discussions. It may be sufficient to reproduce a critical examination of the 1942 Draft Interim Report of the Medical Planning Commission which was published in the British Medical Journal of the 16th January, 1943. This is reproduced in Appendix No. 10.

The principal proposals for the establishment of the National Health Service are summarised as follows in the White Paper: —

Extract from the official Summary of the White Paper

1. *Scope of the New Service.*

   (a) A National Health Service will be established. This service will be available to every citizen in England, Scotland and Wales.

   (b) There will be nothing to prevent those who prefer to make private arrangements for medical attention from doing so. But, for all who wish to use the service it will provide a complete range of personal health care—general and specialist, at home, in the hospital and elsewhere.

(c) The service will be free, apart from possible charges for certain appliances.

2. *Structure of the Service.*

(a) *Central.*

(i) Central responsibility to Parliament and the people will lie with the Minister of Health and the Secretary of State for Scotland.

(ii) At the side of the Minister there will be a professional and expert advisory body to be called the Central Health Services Council. The Council will be a statutory body and its function will be to provide professional guidance on technical aspects of the Health Service. There will be a similar body in Scotland.

(b) *Local.*

Local responsibility will be based on the county and county borough councils, which are the major local government authorities now. They will administer the new service partly in their present separate capacities over their present areas, partly—as the needs of the service require—by combined action in joint boards over larger areas.

At the side of each new joint authority there will be a consultative body—professional and expert—to be called the Local Health Services Council.

Each joint authority will also prepare—in consultation with the Local Health Services Council—and submit for the Minister's approval an "area plan" for securing a comprehensive Health Service of all kinds in its area.

3. *Hospital and Consultant Services.*

It will be the duty of the joint authorities themselves to secure a complete hospital and consultant service for their area—including sanatoria, isolation, mental health services, and ambulance and ancillary services in accordance with the approved area plan.

The joint authorities will do this both by direct provision and by contractual arrangements with voluntary hospitals (or with other joint authorities) as the approved area plan may indicate.

The powers of present local authorities in respect of these services and the ownership of their hospitals will pass to the joint authority.

Consultant services will be made available to all, at the hospitals, local centres, or clinics, or in the home, as required; they will be based on the hospital service, and arranged by the joint authority, either directly or by contact with voluntary hospitals under the approved area plan.

General Medical Practice.

Everyone will be free, under the new Health Service, to choose a doctor—the freedom of choice being limited, as now, only by the number of doctors available and the amount of work which each doctor can properly undertake. Medical practice in the new service will be a combination of grouped and separate practice.

Grouped practice means practice by a group of doctors working in co-operation.

Separate practice means practice by a doctor working on his own account—broadly similar to practice under the present National Health Insurance scheme, but with important changes.

Grouped practice will be conducted normally, though not exclusively, in specially equipped and publicly provided Health Centres. In England and Wales, the Centres will be provided and maintained by county and county borough councils—in Scotland, by the Secretary of State with power to delegate to a local authority.

General practice in the National Health Service will be in the main organised centrally under the responsible Health Ministers. All the main terms and conditions of the doctor's participation will be centrally settled, and much of the day-to-day administration will be the function of Central Medical Boards—one for England and Wales and one for Scotland—largely professional in composition, and acting under the general direction of the Health Ministers.

It is not proposed that there should be a universal salaried system for doctors in the new service. Doctors engaged in Health Centres will be remunerated by salary or the equivalent; doctors in separate practice normally by capitation fee. In some cases—e.g. grouped practice not based on a Health Centre—remuneration by salary or the equivalent could be arranged if the doctors concerned so desired. Rates of remuneration will be discussed with the medical profession.

It is not proposed to prohibit doctors in public practice from engaging also in private practice for any patients who still want this. Where a doctor undertakes private in addition to public practice, the number of patients he is permitted to take under the National Service—and consequently his remuneration—will be adjusted.

Compensation will be paid to any doctor who loses the value of his practice—e.g. by entering a Health Centre or because he is prohibited from transferring the practice to another doctor on the ground that there are too many doctors in the area.

Superannuation schemes will be provided for doctors in Health Centres and the possibility of providing them in other forms of practice will be discussed with the profession, and the practicability of abolishing the sale and purchase of public practices will be similarly discussed.

5. *Clinics and other services.*

It will be the duty of the joint authority to include in its area plan provision for all necessary clinics and other local services (e.g., child welfare, home nursing, health visiting, midwifery and others), and to provide for the co-ordination of these services with the other services in the plan.

6. *Organisation in Scotland.*

The scope and objects of the service will be the same in Scotland as in England and Wales, but subject to certain differences due to special circumstances and the geography and existing local government structure in Scotland.

7. *Finance.*

It is estimated that the cost of the new Service will be about £148,000,000 a year compared with about £61,000,000 spent from public funds on the present health services. The cost will be met from both central and local public funds.

The central expenditure will be direct in the case of the general practitioner service and the State will give grants to local authorities and to voluntary hospitals. How far the central funds will consist of, or be assisted by, sums of money set aside out of contributions under the scheme of national insurance is left over in the White Paper for later consideration.

It is only with the proposals for the general practitioner service that it is necessary for the purposes of this volume to make any extended reference.

Since the publication of the White Paper, the Minister of Health has been in active consultation with the representatives of the medical profession. Although the results of the negotiations have not been published and may doubtless require some further review owing to the election of a new Government, it may be anticipated that, subject to some changes in detail in the proposed central and local administration structure, to the provision of ample safeguards to ensure that any member of the community should be entitled to obtain his medical treatment privately, and to the reservation of the views of the doctors to proposals as regards remuneration and compensation, when these should be set out in the Government plans, the medical profession is prepared to work the new service and to give it their full support.

The repeated declarations in the past of the strong objections of the medical profession to a national service available to everyone in the country, regardless of income, leading eventually, as it has been suggested to the ultimate disappearance of private practice, can be appreciated. But it may fairly be assumed that by now the majority of doctors recognize the inevitability of accepting what is set out in the White Paper. "The new service is designed to provide, for everyone who wishes to use it, a full range of health care. No one will be compelled to use it. Those who prefer to make their own arrangements for medical attention must be free to do so."

Here is what the White Paper has to say about the principles of a general practitioner service: —

"The arrangements for general medical practice are the most important part of the proposals for a National Health Service. The family doctor is the first line of defence in the fight for good health; it is to him that every citizen using the new service will look for advice on his own health and the health of his family; and it is generally through him that access will be had to the many other forms of medical care which the National Service will provide. If there is to be that high degree of confidence between doctor and patient on which the success of the new scheme will depend, two principles must be observed.

First, everyone must be free to choose the doctor whom he consults. Absolute freedom of choice is, of course, impracticable and does not exist now; the number of doctors in any one neighbourhood is necessarily limited. But there must be freedom to choose from among the doctors available.

Second, there must be no such regimentation in the scheme as will prevent a doctor from exercising his professional skill in whatever way he believes to be in the best interests of his patient. Yet, if the State is to provide a universal service of family doctors, there must be some degree of State intervention. The Government believe that their proposals preserve the right degree of balance in this."

Grouped practice and Health Centres.

Under this heading the most significant of the proposals for a general practitioner service is set forth in the White Paper.

"The Government propose that the new service shall be based on a combination of grouped practice and of separate practice, side by side. Grouped practices are more likely to be found suitable in densely populated and highly built-up areas and it is there particularly (though not exclusively) that thev circumstances—dark rooms, facilities for minor surgery and will first be started. It will then be possible to watch the development, with the profession, and to decide in the light of experience how far and how fast a change over to this form of practice should be made.

The conception of grouped practice finds its most usual expression in the idea, advocated by the Medical Planning Commission and others, of conducting practice in specially designed and equipped premises where the group can collaborate and share up-to-date resources—the idea of the Health Centre. The Government agree that in this form the advantages of the group system can be most fully realised, though it will also be desirable to encourage grouped practice without special premises. They intend to design the new service so as to give full scope to the Health Centre system.

The design of a Health Centre will provide for individual consulting-rooms, reception and waiting-rooms, simple laboratory work, nursing and secretarial staff, telephone services and other accessories, as well as—in varying degree according to other ancillaries. The object will be to provide doctors with first class premises and equipment and assistance and so give them the best facilities for meeting their patients' needs and saving their own time.

Health Centres will not affect the patient's freedom to employ the doctor of his choice ; he will be equally free to choose his doctor, whether in a Health Centre, in grouped practice outside the Centre, or in separate practice. Nor will the fact that a doctor is practising in a Health Centre mean that he will not visit his patient at home, when required, just as he does now. Each Centre will need to be so planned as to be regarded by patients, not as a complete break with present habit but as a new place at which they can continue, if they wish, to see their own doctor in better equipped surroundings. Alternatively, they must be able, if they prefer it, simply to choose their Centre rather than any particular doctor in it ; and then the Centre's arrangements must be such as to ensure that they are afforded all the proper advice and treatment which they need."

As regards separate practice the proposal in the White Paper is as follows: —

"In this form of practice the general framework of the National Health Insurance scheme will (with important changes from the past) be retained. A doctor in separate practice will engage himself to provide ordinary medical care and treatment to all persons and families accepted by him under the new arrangements. He will work from his own consulting-room and with his own equipment, as he does now, but he will be backed by the new organised service of consultants, specialists, hospitals, laboratories, and clinics of which he will be enabled and expected to make full use for his patients."

Remuneration of doctors and terms of service.

In the White Paper it is recognised that these are matters for discussion with the medical profession. The Government put forward their general proposals:—

"While they do not believe that a universal change to a salaried system is necessary to the efficient development of the service, and do not therefore propose this course, they consider that there will be parts of the new service to which different considerations will apply. It seems to the Government to be fundamental that in Health Centre practice the grouped doctors working together in a Centre should not be in competition for patients and that in this form of practice remuneration on a capitation system would be inappropriate. They therefore propose that doctors practising in Health Centres shall be remunerated by salaries or on some basis other than that of capitation fees, and they will be ready to discuss with the medical profession the precise system that should be adopted and the salary scales that would be appropriate.

It would also be possible, if desired by the doctors themselves, to offer remuneration by salary or on some similar basis to doctors engaged in group practice, even where the practice was not conducted in a Health Centre and, perhaps, in certain circumstances, to doctors engaged in separate practice. Normally, the remuneration of a doctor in separate practice will be based (at it is now in National Health Insurance) on a capitation system, depending on the number of patients whose care he undertakes—the maximum number of patients whose care any one doctor ought to undertake being, of course, suitably regulated."

The detailed proposals for terms of service are for later consideration. But the contract will obviously need to provide:—

(1) for the doctor to give all normal professional advice and services within his proper competence to those whose care he undertakes;

(2) for him to comply with the approved local arrangements for obtaining consultant and specialist and hospital services;

(3) for proper machinery for the hearing of complaints by patients and for the general kind of disciplinary and appeal procedure already familiar in National Health Insurance;

(4) for the observance of reasonable conditions, centrally determined by the profession, respecting certification and other matters which must arise in any publicly organised service.

An efficient superannuation system will be an essential part of the Health Centre organisation.

It is hoped that the great majority of doctors will take part in the new service and, therefore, it is not proposed to prohibit doctors who enter the service from also treating in their private practices any patients who do not desire to take advantage of the new public arrangements.

Sale and purchase of public practices.

The Government have not overlooked the case which can be made for abolishing the sale and purchase of publicly remunerated practices. The abolition would involve great practical difficulty and is not essential to the working of the new service, and the Government intend to discuss the whole matter further with the profession, including any measures which may be needed to prevent the operation of the new public service from itself increasing the capital value of an individual practice, and therefore also the compensation which may later have to be paid.

Finally, it is recognised that the proposals in the White Paper would, in certain cases, destroy the selling value of existing practices, and where this is so compensation will be paid.

(This completes the main text and the Appendices commence on page 188.)

Appendix No. 1

(a) *The Moulding of the Scheme of National Health Insurance.*

(b) *Starting up the Machine.*

(c) *Why Medical Benefit did not extend to Ireland.*

(a) *The Moulding of the Scheme.*

The story of the moulding of this measure of National Health Insurance set out in detail would make an interesting narrative and, incidentally, would require a whole volume to itself. A few notes must suffice.

Arguments which ranged themselves around large questions of principle, including the way in which the scheme was to be administered, by whom it was to be administered, and the related questions of self-government and control, cannot profitably be reviewed after so long a period of time during which the Act has been in operation, even if space permitted; and this is true also of questions of first importance about which there was a good deal of controversy and discussion before the measure was actually introduced into Parliament, such as that of the State contribution, and whether there should be a State guarantee.

The question of the inclusion of death benefits in the National Health Insurance Scheme was naturally examined in the early days at considerable length, and the decision firmly taken that no death benefits should be included in the scheme.

If death benefits were to have been included the collecting societies and industrial insurance companies, whose political power was tremendous, had to be reckoned with. The later question of the admission of industrial insurance societies into the National Health Insurance scheme was governed very largely by the same arguments as those which decided that the death benefits should be excluded from the scheme. If industrial insurance companies did not come in when they wanted to (because they saw an opportunity of extending their membership enormously instead of losing some of their existing members to the Friendly Societies who would be administering the new scheme), they could hardly have been expected to do otherwise than invest the scheme with an atmosphere of hostility—with disastrous results.

But beyond these major questions—which for the most part were settled before the introduction of the measure into Parliament, there remained a group of questions which had to be dealt with as the measure progressed through Parliament; it is, of course, not in Parliament itself that various modifications and transformations are evolved in the first instance, but outside the House, in conferences, in deputations, and in private interviews. A mere statement of some of these questions is a little overwhelming, e.g. the question of the position of women giving up employment on marriage and re-entering employment during widow-hood; this question, and many related questions concerning women, were the subject of manv interviews and correspondence with representatives of women's organizations. Then there were great social questions, championed by the respective parties. The Conservative Party had as their protagonist Worthington Evans, who spent a great deal of time on the National Insurance Bill, and the party was assisted, incidentally, by Alfred Watson, subsequently appointed Government Actuary, who was in the curious position in 1911 of advising, with the consent of both parties, the Government and those who were in opposition to them—an extraordinarily interesting and difficult position, which only a man with the tact and capacity of Watson could handle satisfactorily. Then there were such questions as low paid labour, casual labour, out-workers, etc., in which the representatives of the Labour Party were especially interested and in regard to which many conferences took place. Employments needing special consideration such as the mercantile marine and share-fishermen, came in for a good deal of attention. Special machinery had to be provided for the insurance of serving sailors and soldiers. Provisions had to be inserted for the exclusion from the insurance provisions of certain employments in which ill health and disablement were already provided for, such as employment in the Civil Service or under a Local Authority. Provision had also to be made for excluding by order from the terms of the scheme various part-time employments, the actual definition of these employments being left for consideration in due course by the Departments. Certain exemptions were introduced under the scheme, whereby a person could claim to be omitted from the compulsory provisions of the scheme by reason of the possession of resources. These exempted persons, however, were to be entitled to medical benefit.

With regard to these questions, it may be said at once that, in so far as some of them were concerned, it was only possible to deal with general principles in the body of the Bill, and leave a great deal to be dealt with by the Commissions when they were set up, by means of regulations, orders, and so on. In due course all of them were settled, somehow or other, but it was something of an achievement to get into the various clauses of the Bill even an inclusive recital of the various problems which had to be dealt with in so far as they were not covered by express provision in the Bill. If a solution of the matters of detail arising in regard to these and a hundred other questions had been attempted in the Bill itself, the probability is that the Bill would never have got through Parliament at all.

In the early days of the Insurance Commission, most of these problems found their solution and were incorporated in regulations and orders, and, except for special problems arising, e.g. out of the War and the difficulties of the following industrial situation, it may be said that the scheme, in its broad outlines, stands to-day very much as it did when, after two or three years, following 1911, it really functioned as a measure. One clause in the Bill which has given rise to much searching of heart amongst constitutionalists was known as the Henry the 8th clause and it empowered the Insurance Commissions by order to remove difficulties. This clause proved to be extremely helpful in the final shaping of the measure, to meet difficulties which arose in practice in the first year or two.

(b) Starting up the Machine.

The story of how the National Health Insurance scheme started cannot well be omitted from this record, but here again a few notes only can be attempted. During the passage of the Bill through Parliament—to be exact, I think it was in the autumn of 1911—a wave of sturdy nationalism swept over the House, and, in due course, when the Bill became law, separate Commissions were set up for England, Ireland, Scotland, and Wales. Ireland, of course, began it, and the first demand, as might have been expected, was that Ireland should have been left entirely out of the Bill but that the State contribution towards the scheme should be put into a separate fund for the benefit of the Irish. This, however, did not materialize although, owing to the special circumstances of the medical service in Ireland, the Irish insured persons were excluded from the medical benefit provisions of the Bill. A short account of how the Irish question was treated is contained in part (*c*) of this Appendix.

Ireland having led the way for a national scheme—a demand which was met by the promise to set up a separate Irish Commission—there followed almost immediately a pressing demand from the Scottish members of the House for a separate Scottish Commission; and it is hardly necessary to add that, as a distinguished Welshman had introduced the scheme which was to bear his name all over the country, there followed a demand for a Welsh Insurance Commission. So it came about that before the year 1911 had come to its close, and while the Bill was still before the House of Lords, separate bodies of Commissioners were appointed for England, Ireland, Scotland, and Wales. As it would appear that they were all going to do the same thing more or less in the same way, it was necessary to have a co-ordinating body. Accordingly, the National Health Insurance Joint Committee was set up, consisting of the chairman of each of the four Commissions, with Treasury and other representatives, the whole being under the chairmanship of the responsible Minister. The first Minister was Mr. Charles Masterman.

The first step after the appointment of the Commissions was to expand the very small nucleus of staff which had been engaged upon the Bill while it was passing through Parliament and to create out of it a staff for the National Health Insurance Commission in England under the chairmanship of Sir Robert Morant. The deputy chairman was Dr. Smith Whitaker, the medical secretary of the British Medical Association, and he incurred a great amount of odium amongst his fellow practitioners because of his acceptance of this appointment. As, however, in due course, I worked with Smith Whitaker as his "opposite number" on the secretariat for some years, I can give my personal testimony to the fact that his acceptance of the post of deputy chairman of the Insurance Commission was definitely taken in the public interest and in the interests of the medical profession. So far from being a traitor to his fellows, the step which he took was designed to bring about—and succeeded in this respect—a very much better understanding between the medical profession and the administrative body, and led, in due course, to the medical profession having a steadily increasing share in the actual administration of the scheme.

Staffing and office accommodation were obviously the first steps for the Commissions to consider, and, looking back at the men who were roped in for the great adventure, and also to their subsequent careers, one may fairly say that it was indeed a Ministry of all the talents. A mere recital of the names of a great many of the distinguished civil servants who took part in this great adventure— amongst them Sir John Anderson and Sir Arthur Salter—would be impressive.

The outcome of this sturdy wave of nationalism resulted, of course, in a very heavy expenditure on administration out of proportion to the results secured. There were, naturally, some problems of detail affecting Ireland or Scotland or Wales, which could best be dealt with by people on the spot, but, in the main, the scheme was one for the whole of the United Kingdom, and the provisions which were adopted by the English Commission were closely followed, in due course, by the other Commissions as far as the circumstances would permit. It was no doubt of great advantage to have meetings in London of the National Health Insurance Joint Committee, and to have the representatives' points of view duly put forward by the chairmen of the several Commissions, but it is really difficult to suppose that this result could not equally have been obtained by having one central body in London with staffs in Edinburgh, Cardiff, and Dublin.

(c) *Why Medical Benefit did not extend to Ireland.*

Extract from the Carmichael Prize Essay of 1913, by Mr. H. Nelson Hardy, F.R.C.S., Edinburgh.

(In this extract Mr. Hardy relates how it came to pass that Ireland was left out of the Bill so far as medical benefits were concerned).

About the same time that the Irish College of Physicians had considered the subject, and passed the resolutions (previously quoted), the Roman Catholic hierarchy in Ireland held an important meeting at Maynooth, and passed a resolution asking the Chancellor of the Exchequer not to extend the Bill to Ireland, but to set aside the State contribution necessary for financing the scheme to the credit of Ireland, either for an insurance scheme to be specially devised for the needs of Ireland, or for some other purpose that might be deemed more beneficial to the general welfare of the population; and they called upon the Irish Nationalist Party to urge this policy in Parliament. They based their argument on the statement that while the Bill might do for England and Wales, of which 78 per cent. of the inhabitants are urban and only 22 per cent. rural, it did not suit a country like Ireland, of whose population only 28 per cent. are urban and 72 per cent. rural, and of whom only a mere fraction—either urban or rural—are wage earners, the immense majority being workers on their own account, such as farmers, shop-keepers, and others, who neither receive nor pay wages. They stated further that in their opinion the measure would increase unemployment. There can be little doubt, however, adds the medical reporter to *The Lancet*, that among other things influencing the prelates was the well-known fact that the small farmers and their wives and children, who work on the land, can always at present obtain gratuitous medical attendance and medicines through the widespread dispensary system, which has no parallel in either England or Scotland. The result was that, through the influence of Mr. Redmond and his party, Ireland was ultimately left out of the scheme so far as regards medical benefits.

Appendix No. 2

INDUSTRIAL ASSURANCE.

All offices : Companies and Collecting Societies.

Year	Growth of Business			
	Premiums Received £	Funds at end of Year £	Expenses of Management £	Ratio of Expenses to Prems. %
1877 ..	*2,036,135	1,802,065		
1887 ..	*5,316,920	8,494,983		
1897 ..	*9,511,196	21,461,640		
1907 ..	*17,042,108	47,730,206		
1917 ..	25,174,082	83,445,578	10,264,294	40·77
1922 ..	38,668,405	133,919,997	15,763,014	40·76
1927 ..	48,050,747	217,106,714	16,552,407	34·45
1932 ..	57,332,230	296,392,622	19,080,418	33·28
1935 ..	63,725,885	360,614,639	21,984,435†	34·50
1936 ..	66,394,557	385,063,491	22,409,497†	33·75

* These figures include interest and other miscellaneous income for Collecting Societies.

† After 1932 the Commissioner's return of Expenses includes appropriations of surplus to Staff bonuses and staff superannuation funds.

The figures for 1917 and onwards for Premiums received, Funds and Expenses of Management are taken from the Industrial Assurance Commissioner's Annual Reports or Statistical Summaries. The figures prior to 1917 are taken from Kelham and Levey on "Some recent developments on Industrial Assurance in Great Britain," a paper read to the Eighth International Congress of Actuaries.

The following figures show the amount of business "in force" under Whole Life Assurances and Endowments and Endowment Assurances at specified valuations.

Year	Whole Life			Endowment and Endowment Assurance		
	Number	Sums Assured £	Average Sum Assured per policy £	Number	Sums Assured	Average Sum Assured per policy £
1925 ..	56,827,353	738,926,834	13·00	9,254,174	236,805,285	25·59
1930 ..	62,079,752	894,802,212	14·41	7,756,620	199,062,626	25·66
1935 ..	66,764,183	1,024,725,103	15·35	9,602,662	254,880,116	26·54

The information is taken from the Reports of the Industrial Assurance Commissioner: the three years in question are the only ones where it is possible to obtain complete figures as the usual practice for Societies is to value quinquennially.

APPENDIX NO. 3

STATISTICS OF REGISTERED PROVIDENT SOCIETIES

EXTRACT FROM GENERAL SUMMARY PUBLISHED BY THE

CHIEF REGISTRAR OF FRIENDLY SOCIETIES

ON 22nd JULY, 1937.

Explanatory Notes.

The general summary contains statistical information extracted from the returns of all societies and other bodies on the register and also of industrial assurance companies.

The figures for funds have been compiled so as to represent as nearly as possible the combined savings of the members, i.e., the total sums accumulated in specific funds for the collective benefit of the members, or the aggregate of the amounts standing to their credit in shares, deposits, etc., as the case may be.

In preparing the totals of the various groups in the summary a considerable amount of duplication necessarily arises in the figures for membership and funds. A person may be a member of more than one society, e.g., he may be a member of a friendly society, a co-operative society and a trade union, be a shareholder in a building society and also hold one or more policies in an industrial assurance office. It is not possible in combining the membership figures to attempt any elimination of this duplication. In compiling the funds, however, adjustments have been made, so far as is practicable, to eliminate duplication due to inter-investment and dual registration.

Detailed statistics for friendly societies, industrial and provident societies, trade unions and building societies will be found in Parts 2, 3, 4 and 5 respectively of the Chief Registrar's Report. For collecting and industrial assurance companies, detailed statistics are given in the Report of the Industrial Assurance Commissioner.

	No. of Societies on Register at end of year			No. of Members 000's			Total Fund £000's		
	1913	1925	1935	1913	1925	1935	1913	1925	1935
Friendly Societies Acts—									
(1) Friendly Societies ..	25,475	22,777	20,245	6,783	7,252	8,201	51,489	86,533	135,312
(2) Other Societies	2,509	2,571	2,704	709	973	1,038	2,488	4,640	6,772
Industrial Assurance—									
(3) Collecting Societies ..	71	182	151	(6)7,481	(6)15,423	(6)22.807	11,165	33,668	69,577
Companies	19	18	15	(6)37,556	(6)55,288	(6)71,035	55,762	151,785	296,712
Industrial and Provident Societies	3,086	5,904	5,691	3,208	5,900	8,610	53,634	122,545	(8)250,055
Building Societies	1,551	1,092	999	617	1,129	1,939	65,316	164,135	592,634
Trade Unions	616	579	537	3,220	4,492	3,851	6,507	12,717	14,478
(4) Workmen's Compensation Schemes	23	17	10	74	57	45	69	50	33
Certified Loan Societies ..	249	131	102	31	23	21	235	192	163
Railway Savings Banks ..	19	12	10	76	154	161	7,427	15,044	23,100
(5) Superannuation and Other Trust Funds	—	—	254	—	—	(7) —	—	—	65,674
Total	33,618	33,283	30,718	59,755	90,691	117,708	254,082	589,758	1,442,935

(1) Includes Friendly Societies with Branches (" Orders ").

(2) Working Men's Clubs, Specially Authorised Societies, etc.

(3) Registered under the Friendly Societies Acts. Figures include business in respect of benefit funds other than Industrial.

(4) Excludes the Admiralty, War Office and Air Ministry Scheme.

(5) Registered under the Superannuation and other Trust Funds (Validation) Act, 1927.

(6) Assurances or policies.

(7) Not available.

(8) For 1935, includes loans from members. The amount so brought in is £31,580,000. In previous years such loans have been omitted

APPENDIX No. 4

MEMORANDUM (1926) WITH REGARD TO THE FINANCIAL QUESTIONS EXAMINED IN THE REPORT OF THE ROYAL COMMISSION ON NATIONAL HEALTH INSURANCE.

1. It it not easy to get a clear perspective of the several financial questions examined by the Commission, partly because they are to be sought in different sections of the Report, and partly because the amounts involved are stated sometimes in figures of cost per annum and at other times in fractions of a penny of the weekly contribution. It is proposed therefore in this note to set out the principal financial considerations quite broadly and to express the amounts concerned in a uniform way (cost in pounds per annum for the whole insured population) so that they may be considered in relation to one another.

2. A useful figure to keep in mind is that there are 15 million insured persons in Great Britain, and that an expenditure of 1/- per head per annum on any benefit is equivalent to a sum of £750,000 per annum.

3. The questions reviewed will be dealt with under three heads

(a) Existing surpluses of Approved Societies;

(b) The margin in the present weekly contribution;

(c) The cost of extensions of benefits.

(a) *Existing Surpluses of Approved Societies.*

4. These are the amounts which, on a valuation made by the Government Actuary every five years, are found to be available to the Approved Societies for expenditure on additional benefits. In the valuation, the Actuary makes full provision for all statutory reserves but, having declared a surplus, he recommends that a part of it should be carried forward to a future valuation, and the remainder only spent on additional benefits. These "additional benefits" are under the control of the Approved Societies, and are not enjoyed by the whole insured population;

some Societies have large surpluses; others have small surpluses or none at all; others have a deficiency.

5. The surpluses declared at the end of the first five-yearly period amounted to 17 million pounds, of which 9 millions was applied to additional benefits, and 8 millions carried forward. With regard to this valuation, the Commissioners state that, owing to the disturbing factor of the war, they did not feel justified in making any general assumption from the fact of so large a surplus.

6. The second valuation is not quite complete, but it is stated that, including sums carried forward from the previous valuation (with their subsequent interest earnings) the surpluses are expected to amount to between 40 millions and 45 millions, of which it is estimated that 15 millions will be carried forward, and 25-30 millions applied to additional benefits.

7. The amount applicable under the second valuation to additional benefits, spread over a five-yearly period, is therefore equivalent to an expenditure of 5 to 6 millions a year.

8. Since the second valuation, further large surpluses are stated to have accrued, estimated to amount, by the end of the year 1926, to a sum well in excess of 35 million pounds—including the carry-forward of 15 millions from the second valuation—leaving a sum of probably 20 millions as the surplus currently accumulating in a period of three years (from 31st December, 1923, to 31st December, 1926), say, 7 millions a year.

9. As to all these accrued surpluses, it is recommended that no part of them should be applied to extensions of statutory benefits. They will be used, so far as they are not required to be carried forward to a later valuation—for such "additional benefits" as the Societies, subject to the general guidance of the Ministry, think fit.

(b) The Margin in the Weekly Contribution.

10. The existence of these large surpluses has led the Commission, with the assistance of an actuarial committee, to consider whether the present weekly health insurance contributions are not too high. The main causes of the surpluses are the high rate of interest which is being earned on all balances in insurance funds, and the lower rates of sickness which have obtained, compared

with the expectation. The low sickness rate is, however, subject to what are referred to as disquieting features, in the course of the claims from year to year, especially among women and in regard to their claims for disablement benefit.

11. The weekly contribution has, in fact, already been reduced this year, mainly because of the transfer, from Health Insurance funds to Pension funds, of the claims of persons between 65 and 70 years of age. Apart from this reduction, the Commission find that there is a margin in the contributions amounting (with the equivalent Exchequer grant) to 4½ million pounds a year, in other words, 4½ million pounds more is being raised than is necessary to meet the anticipated expenditure on current statutory benefits. The margin, in terms of the weekly contribution, is not sufficient for it to be practicable to recommend a reduction in the contribution itself, and it is, moreover, unequally distributed between men and women; (the excess is 7/- per head per annum in the case of men and 3/9d. in the case of women).

12. The way in which this margin is proposed to be used can be briefly stated. Medical benefit costs 12/6d. per head per annum (that is £9,375,000). Of this amount 9/6d. (£7,125,000) is already a permanent statutory charge on insurance funds, and a balance of 3/- (£2,250,000) has been met by temporary provision for three years under an Act of 1924. It is proposed that this balance of 2¼ millions should now be met out of the margin so that the whole cost of medical benefit will become a normal statutory charge on insurance funds.

13. As to the remainder of the margin of 4½ million pounds, amounting to 2¼ million pounds a year, although the method of applying this to a scheme for extra sickness allowance for workers with dependants is examined in the Report, there is a pretty clear hint* that the whole sum will in fact go to the relief of the

*Since this Memorandum was written, the Economy Bill has appeared with its accompanying explanatory note. This shows that the Exchequer is appropriating this sum and that in fact the Exchequer saving on National Health Insurance will be 2¾ million pounds per annum. This is half a million pounds in excess of the figure of the Exchequer saving referred to in paragraph 13. It is perhaps sufficient for the purpose of this Memorandum to say that the Exchequer relief provided by the Economy Bill takes the form of a reduction of the fraction which represents that part of the cost of all benefits borne by the Exchequer. This fractional reduction extends not only to the normal statutory benefits, but to the additional benefits, which have now reached very considerable proportions. The Exchequer saving on the latter may well be at least ½ million of money, and the figure in paragraph 13 of 2¼ million may therefore stand as relating to the normal statutory benefits. This means that the estimate of future surpluses referred to in paragraph 17 need not be disturbed.

Exchequer contribution (to the cost of benefits generally) under the Insurance Acts. No part of the margin in that case will be available for extensions of the statutory benefits.

(*c*) *Cost of Extensions of Benefits.*

14. The cost of extended services is not therefore to be met out of past surpluses, nor out of the margin of the weekly contributions.

15. The recommendation made by the Commission for a scheme of extended medical services is placed first in order of priority. They state that whether the cost is to be met in the way they recommend, or in some other way, such extension should receive first and immediate consideration.

16. The method recommended for meeting the cost is the pooling of one-half of the future surpluses* of the Societies.

17. The sum proposed to be subject to this pooling is the amount of the surpluses hereafter earned from year to year, and does not include any balances brought forward from any earlier period or even the interest on such balances. The amount of the new surpluses (so limited) is assumed by the Commission to be 2 million pounds a year. This is doubtless a conservative estimate. The surplus under existing conditions appears to be about 7 million pounds per annum (see paragraph 8). The amount proposed to be applied out of future contributions, as stated in paragraphs 12-13, is 4½ millions per annum. If this is regarded as reducing future surpluses and is deducted from 7 million pounds per annum, it leaves 2½ million a year as an esti-

* Notwithstanding the using up of the available "margin" in the weekly contributions, as explained in pars. 12-13, surpluses will continue to arise. The actuaries must assume a general level—and a fairly high general level—of sickness benefit for the scheme as a whole, and they calculate that certain contributions are required to pay that benefit. But the scheme is administered by Societies with widely differing experiences, and many—a considerable number—may still be expected to have surpluses, while some of course will be in a deficiency. The alternative, i.e. if the actuaries assumed a lower general level of sickness, would be that a large number of societies would show a deficiency. As it is, the Actuarial Advisory Committee anticipates that Societies representing 10 per cent. of the insured population will be in a deficiency under the new basis of calculation (and provision is made for assisting such Societies).

This aspect of the case must be borne in mind in looking for a motive for the Commission's recommendation to pay for extensions of benefit out of future surpluses. The alternative method, of charging the costs against the normal funds, woud throw a much larger number of Societies into deficiency, although the burden, spread over the whole of the insurance funds, and for a number of years, would ultimately be the same.

mate of current surpluses under the new conditions. The Commission say 2 million pounds a year, but they recognise that it is impossible to make any precise estimate. Their recommendation is that half of this amount should be pooled. This half would be equal to a sum of one million pounds a year on the Commission's assumption, or 1¼ millions on the alternative calculation.

18. The estimated maximum cost of the new services recommended is as follows: —

Specialist services	£940,000
Bedside consultations	£250,000
Laboratory aids...	£100,000
	£1,290,000

These figures, however, are for England and Wales, and the cost of the services for Great Britain as a whole is stated in round figures at 1½ million pounds per annum. On the above proportions the cost of services for Great Britain may roughly be stated as follows: —

Specialist services	£1,100,000
Bedside consultations...	£290,000
Laboratory aids	£110,000
	£1,500,000

19. It is of interest to note that, notwithstanding their estimate of one million pounds as representing one-half of future surpluses, the Commission state elsewhere, with regard to the cost of the new services, which they place at 1½ million pounds per annum, that "the money can be obtained by such a scheme of pooling as we have proposed".

It is possible that they had in mind the gradual bringing into the general insurance pool of certain special reserves of the kind which have been temporarily drawn upon for three years only under the Act of 1924 towards the current cost of Medical Benefit.

CONCLUSIONS.

20. The Commission's financial conclusions (as modified by the Economy Bill) can therefore be shortly stated as follows: —

(*a*) No part of the surpluses already accrued—whether available for "additional benefits," or carried forward to a future valuation—is to be applied to the extension of statutory services.

(*b*) The weekly Health Insurance contribution is higher than is necessary to provide for existing statutory benefits, but the excess will be absorbed (i) in making full provision for the cost of existing medical benefit, and (ii) in the relief of the Exchequer contributions to the Insurance Schemes as a whole.

(*c*) The cost of the extensions of Medical Benefit, estimated at 1½ millions per annum, can be met out of one-half of the future surpluses of the Approved Societies.

21. It may be added that the pooling of half of the surpluses would appear to make adequate provision for the new services as above valued, but no more. It may be assumed that the extended services could be brought into operation as soon as the administrative arrangements permit, and could be financed provisionally by advances out of insurance funds generally, repayments being made in due course out of the half-surpluses when they have been ascertained at the next valuation.

Appendix No. 5

Extract from the Report by the Government Actuary on the Fourth Valuation of the Assets and Liabilities of Approved Societies.

On the present occasion the valuations have been made on the basis prescribed by the National Health Insurance (Valuation) Regulations, 1933. Under these regulations the future claims for sickness and disablement benefits are estimated, in the case of men, to be in close accordance with the rates of sickness shown by the Manchester Unity Experience, 1893-97; this involves no change from the rates employed in the third valuation. In the case of women, however, the actuarial basis was revised in connection with the National Health Insurance and Contributory Pensions Act, 1932, and the rates of sickness then adopted have been used for the present valuations. The new basis was provided by the experience in the three years 1928-30 of a group of societies, so selected as to be typical of the whole. For reasons explained in the next paragraph, rates of sickness were determined for unmarried and married women respectively, which were financially equivalent, in the aggregate, to 90 per cent of the rates exhibited by that experience. Further, the assumed proportion of women who remain in employment after marriage was increased from one-seventh to one-fifth.

The alterations in the provision for sickness, disablement and maternity claims in the case of women were made at the same time as the reduction, under the Act of 1932, in the rates of disablement benefit for unmarried women from 7s. 6d. to 6s. a week, and in the rates of sickness and disablement benefits for married women from 12s. and 7s. 6d. to 10s. and 5s. a week respectively. In the case of unmarried women the new provision allows, on the average, for 15 per cent. more weeks of sickness benefit and 100 per cent. more weeks of disablement benefit than would result if the basis employed for men were used to assess the claims of this class: in the case of married women the corresponding additions to the provision are about 130 per cent. and 205 per cent. for sickness and disablement benefits respectively.

Taking the combined benefits, the cost provided for is greater by approximately 35 per cent. in respect of unmarried women, and 150 per cent. in respect of married women, than it would have been if the rates of incapacity applicable to men had been employed.

In conjunction, the several modifications amounted to a financial reconstruction of women's insurance, so arranged as to preserve the principle that, on the basis of valuation adopted, the contributions credited to the benefit fund of a society should be equivalent in value to the related benefits and cost of administration in the case of an entrant into insurance at the age of 16. The financial effect of the changes was explained in the Report by the Government Actuary on the Financial Provisions of the National Health Insurance and Contributory Pensions Bill, 1932 (Cmd. 4073), from which it will be observed that the equivalence of benefits (at the rates fixed in the Bill) and contributions was only secured on the assumption that the rates of sickness would be maintained at a level 10 per cent. lower on average than that of the years 1928-30.

Appendix No. 6

Percentage of weeks of Sickness to "Expectation," Years 1921-7.

Year	Men		Women			
			Unmarried		Married	
	Sickness Benefit	Disablement Benefit	Sickness Benefit	Disablement Benefit	Sickness Benefit	Disablement Benefit
1921	76	54	73	60	63	66
1922	89	65	88	67	82	73
1923	86	72	91	77	92	90
1924	97	81	105	86	110	104
1925	98	83	112	99	121	125
1926	108	93	112	111	124	146
1927	107	100	117	119	130	171

It will be seen from this statement that in respect of each ot the three classes of insured persons the claims for both sickness benefit and disablement benefit have been rising continuously during the seven years. Comparing 1927 with 1921 the following results are brought out:

Sickness Benefit.

The claims of men have risen by ... ... 41 per cent.
" " unmarried women have risen by 60 "
" " married women have risen by 106 "

Disablement Benefit.

The claims of men have risen by ... ... 85 per cent.
" " unmarried women have risen by 100 "
" " married women have risen by 159 "

It is evident from the Table that in the early years of the period the moderation of the claims was a factor of substantial importance in the production of valuation surpluses. Since 1926 in the case of men, and 1924 in the case of women, the position in this respect has undergone a serious change.

APPENDIX No. 7

EXTRACTS FROM REPORTS OF MEDICAL SERVICE SUB-COMMITTEE (London Insurance Committee)

Cases considered by the Medical Service Sub-Committee mainly relate to—

(1) Irregular certification by insurance practioners, in which event the complainant is usually the Approved Society concerned;

(2) Treatment, whether as to failure to provide, as to negligence or, occasionally, a failure to diagnose a particular condition (ordinarily a question of diagnosis is not a question to be considered by the Sub-Committee provided the practitioner has examined the insured person and has formed an honest opinion as to his condition)

(3) Improperly charging fees to insured persons.

Failure to provide treatment.

CASE A. A practitioner received a telephone call at 8-30 a.m. from the mistress of the insured person. He asked whether the case was urgent and on receiving a reply in the negative said that he thought it was confounded impertinence to ring up a doctor at 8-30 a.m. about a panel call. The mistress told him that if that was his attitude towards the case he need not call and that she would obtain the services of another doctor, which she did. The practitioner called later on in the day but was not permitted to see the patient. The Committee were of opinion that the complaint had been substantiated, they deprecated the practitioner's conduct very strongly and warned him that the expression used by him was open to the interpretation that his attitude of mind towards his practice among insured persons was prejudicial to the service and might, if persisted in, entail serious consequences.

CASE B. An insured person returned home from work on Christmas Eve and complained of not feeling well. By the evening of Christmas Day his temperature had risen to 101°, and at about 7.15 p.m. his mother went to the practitioner's house to ask for a visit. She was seen by a manservant, who said that the practitioner would be available at 12 o'clock noon on the following day. On Boxing Day the parents expected a visit, but as the practitioner did not call and the patient's temperature had risen to 103° his father telephoned the practitioner at about 10 o'clock p.m. After some argument, the practitioner said he was not satisfied that the case was one of urgency but would call the following morning. The father told the practitioner that he regarded this as a refusal to call that night; that he would call in another doctor and the practitioner need not call on the following morning. Expenses amounting to £1 13s. 6d. were entailed as a result. The practitioner was cautioned; he was required to repay the amount expended in obtaining treatment from another doctor and, in due course, the sum of £2 was withheld from his remuneration.

CASE C. A domestic servant was severely burned and telephonic application was made for the services of the practitioner concerned. He advised removal to hospital, but made no attempt to visit the patient or to facilitate her admission to hospital. He was censured and the Committee requested the Minister to withhold £20 from his remuneration.

CASE D. A man of 65 years of age suffering from bronchitis and cardiac debility, was under treatment by a practitioner's assistant from January to March, but during that time only four visits were made to him and then only after specific requests. On one occasion following a visit on a Sunday a week elapsed without any further attendance by the assistant and on the following Saturday the man's wife went to the surgery and asked the assistant to call. As he had not visited by Monday, she went again to the surgery and he called the same day. At the wife's request the man was sent to hospital on 28th March and died there a week later. It appeared to the Sub-Committee in their consideration of the case that there was running right through it evidence of a failure to provide that standard of treatment which is required and expected of insurance practitioners. The practitioner had to accept responsibility for the acts of the assistant whose conduct was described as censurable and the sum of £10 was withheld.

Certification.

CASE E. An insured person was discharged from hospital on 4th April and on that day he presented to the Society a certificate covering the period during which he was an in-patient. On 12th June the insured person went to the practitioner and obtained from him four intermediate certificates dated respectively 16th, 23rd and 30 May and 7th June. The insured person had some weeks earlier obtained a duplicate of his discharge certificate from the hospital and attempted to impose it upon the Society with a view to obtaining a second payment of benefit but without success. The insured person was then committed to prison but on his release took the duplicate hospital certificate to the practitioner and requested and obtained the four certificates referred to above. The irregular certificates were used by the insured person in an attempt to obtain benefit from the Society but again his application was unsuccessful. The practitioner's excuse was that when the insured person consulted him on 12th June he was of opinion that the patient was incapable of work by reason of "weakness through diabetes", and that he had been incapacitated during the period covered by the certificates. He felt that the insured person should not, owing to ignorance, lose the benefit to which the practitioner thought he was entitled and he accordingly took upon himself the responsibility of issuing the certificates. The report of the Medical Service Sub-Committee says that they did not allow the picturesque touch which is given to this case by the insured person's sojourn in gaol to influence their recommendation, but it served to illustrate somewhat vividly the interesting possibilities where a practitioner ignores the clear requirements of the certification rules and the meaning of the King's English. The practitioner was warned of the necessity for strict adherence to the Medical Certification Rules and £10 was withheld from his remuneration.

CASE F. An insured person had been under the medical care of the practitioner for five years, suffering with cardiac trouble and cataleptic fits. About two and a half years before the case was heard by the Medical Service Sub-Committee the patient was seen by the practitioner in consultation with an R.M.O. and the latter expressed the view that nothing more could be done for the patient by way of medical treatment. Shortly afterwards the practitioner arranged for a specialist with whom he was acquainted to see the patient and as a result she was admitted to a hospital and remained there for a considerable time. On her discharge the practitioner was informed that nothing more could be done for the patient and since that time he had not seen her but had been furnished each month by her mother with a report, and on these reports he issued certificates of incapacity stating that the insured person was rendered incapable of work by reason of endocarditis. This practice had been in operation for a period of over a year and a half and in each of the certificates the practitioner had certified that he had examined the insured person on the date appended to the certificate. The practitioner told the Sub-Committee that the case had exceptional features in that the insured person was suffering from major hysteria and was mentally affected. He knew that by visiting the patient she became excited and that this would do her more harm than good and it was this reason which influenced him in not going to see her. The practitioner was warned and the sum of £5 recommended to be withheld from his remuneration.

Fee Charging.

CASE G. Two practitioners in partnership had a general waiting room and another waiting room approached by a private door, and complaint was made that insured persons who entered the general waiting room were required to wait a long while, while others who paid a fee for admission to the private waiting room received preferential treatment. The senior partner told the Medical Service Sub-Committee that he had acquired the practice some twenty-three years before and that at the time he took the practice over it had been the custom for patients who entered by the side door to pay a fee of one shilling a week whilst under treatment for the privilege of waiting in the room to which the side door led. The practitioner stated emphatically that no differentiation whatever was made in the treatment provided and that so far as he could ascertain the only reason why patients preferred to go to the side door and not to wait in the general waiting room was that they thereby avoided waiting in the company of people with whom perhaps they did not wish to sit. The practice of accepting these fees had obtained ever since he had taken over the practice notwithstanding the fact that he joined the Medical List in January, 1913. Asked what would happen if an insured patient, who was not aware of the custom prevailing in the practice, went to the side door he said that the patient would be told that he should not go to that door unless the case was urgent. He would treat the patient and tell him that if he desired to use the side door in future he would have to pay an extra shilling per week for the privilege. The practitioner and his partner had over three thousand insured persons included in their list at the time of the hearing of the case, and the Committee took a serious view of the breach of the Terms of Service which the practitioner had committed by accepting for over ten years fees from insured persons in the circumstances indicated. Both practitioners were severely censured; they were required to give the Committee an assurance that the practice of charging for admission to the side door would not be reverted to and in due course the sum of £150 was withheld from their remuneration.

Refusal to visit a patient.

CASE H. An insured person stated that having been discharged from a hospital and becoming ill on the same evening, she caused a message to be sent to an insurance practitioner on the following morning requesting a home visit. The practitioner declined to attend and she accordingly secured the services of another practitioner incurring thereby expenses amounting to 5/-. The practitioner's reply was to the effect that on the afternoon of the day on which the patient was discharged from hospital he received a telephone call from the House Physician to one of the Honorary Staff there to the effect that the patient had discharged herself voluntarily; that she had been in bed for two weeks, had been examined by the member of the Honorary Staff personally, had had numerous X-rays taken and every conceivable pathological test all with negative result. The hospital authorities had told her that she was not ill, but had advised her to remain a day longer in order to get used to being out of bed. She had, however, discharged herself—he had attended her either at her home or at his surgery forty-three times during the previous year without ever finding any signs of physical disease. He agreed with the opinion of the House Physician that whilst there might be a neurotic element in the patient's condition she was not physically ill. On the following morning he received a clinical report from the hospital and soon afterwards received a message from the patient's mother asking him to visit the patient. He was engaged with another patient at the time and accordingly sent a message that he had been informed by the hospital that the patient was not ill and that if she wished to see him she could call at his surgery, which was less than two minutes' walk from her home. The mother sent a further message that her daughter was ill and wished him to call, to which he replied that he was then engaged but would be prepared to see the mother herself in half an hour. No further attempt was made to obtain his services. The insured person submitted a certificate from the other practitioner whom she called in to the effect that when he visited her he found her suffering from a febrile attack with pain in her back, vomiting, headache and general malaise and that he did not consider her fit to leave home on that occasion. The Sub-Committee found that there was no failure on the part of the practitioner to comply with the Terms of Service for Insurance Practitioners.

Appendix No. 8.

A SHORT HISTORICAL NOTE ON THE CAPITATION SYSTEM OF PAYMENT, AND OF THE METHOD BY WHICH THE DOCTORS' REMUNERATION WAS FORMERLY CALCULATED.

(i) *The amount of the capitation fee.*

In calculations made for the purpose of the Insurance Bill in 1911, 6/- per head of the insured population was estimated as the cost of Medical Benefit, including both treatment and medicine. It soon became clear that this was not regarded by the medical profession as adequate. After lengthy negotiations the amount was increased to 9/-. Out of this sum of 9/-, 2/- was set aside as a drug fund, and 7/- for the doctors' professional services. The doctors, however, had an interest in the 2/- drug fund, whereby, if the cost of the drugs in any area fell below an average of 2/- a head, the difference up to a maximum of 6d. a head was added to the remuneration of the doctors in the area. This came to be known as the "floating sixpence" and its effect was that the average capitation fee before the War was about 7/3d. The arrangement was abolished as from the 1st January, 1920.

During the War, and for some time after, certain additional payments were made to doctors. From 1917 onwards accounts for treatment given to invalid ex-service men were paid, even though the amounts exceeded what would be produced by the 9/- capitation fee, but subject to some slight discount; and certain war bonuses were paid in the years 1918 and 1919.

Early in the year 1920, after prolonged discussion between the doctors and the Government, the question of remuneration was referred to arbitration and the capitation fee was fixed at 11/-, as against the pre-war capitation fee of about 7/3d. It was agreed on both sides that the finding of the arbitrators should be accepted for at least a year, and it was, in fact, observed to the end of the year 1921.

In addition to the capitation fee of 11/-, a special mileage fund was set up for the purpose of making an extra payment to all doctors who practise in rural and semi-rural areas. Before the year 1920, there had been only a mileage fund of a comparatively small amount for making payments in areas where the travelling was exceptionally difficult.

At the beginning of the year 1922,* the capitation fee was reduced from 11/- to 9/6d., the general arrangements in regard to the constitution of the mileage fund being continued. It was decided that the new capitation fee of 9/6d. should continue in force for a period of two years, that is, to the end of the year 1923. The Minister then offered 8/- for five years, or 8/6d. for three years. This was refused and resignations were handed in by over 90 per cent. of the insurance practitioners. The Minister then offered to pay 8/6d. for five years, or to refer the matter to an independent Court of Inquiry, and the doctors accepted the latter alternative. The decision of the Court was for a capitation fee of 9/-.

(ii) *Earlier methods of calculation.*

The method of calculating each doctor's remuneration, which was in force up to the year 1920, was as follows: —

As soon as possible after the end of each year, the total number of insured persons for that year was ascertained by counting the number of contribution cards (that is, cards to which the weekly insurance stamps are affixed) given up by the insured population. The number so ascertained was multiplied by the capitation fee of 9/- and the amount paid into a central pool. Out of this pool was set aside the amount required for drugs, and the balance was distributed amongst the insurance committees for the counties and county boroughs in proportion to their respective insured populations as shown by the counts of their registers. This sum was then distributed locally amongst the doctors, the necessary adjustments having first been made in regard to the "floating sixpence," already referred to, and other corrections having been made for movements, between one area and another, of persons temporarily absent from home.

Experience, however, showed that, owing to the delay in the surrendering of contribution cards and the difficulty of securing

* The reduction of the capitation fee from 11/- to 9/6d. was accepted by insurance practitioners at this time under the assurance and in the belief that national circumstances necessitated a sacrifice.

accurate and punctual information as to the movements of the insured population from one area to another, the calculation of the central pool and its distribution to insurance committees could not be made until long after the close of the year, and delays in the final settlement of the payment to doctors were a constant source of irritation to them. Moreover, changes made in the insurance scheme affecting persons who ceased to pay contributions, by which such persons continued for a time to be entitled to medical benefit, rendered necessary some modification of the contribution card basis for ascertaining the number of persons entitled to medical treatment. A new method (see page 155) of procedure was therefore evolved and brought into operation as from the beginning of 1920.

Appendix No. 9.

THE SUMS AVAILABLE FOR MEDICAL BENEFIT.

The question of the sums available for the cost of Medical Benefit, and the sources from which they flow, can only be considered as a whole, i.e., to include payment to chemists as well as to doctors.

In 1911, the financial scheme of the National Insurance Bill included a sum of 6/- per head of the insured population for Medical Benefit (doctors and chemists). This was to come, as to seven-ninths from the contributions of the employed person and his employer, and two-ninths from the Exchequer. After negotiations with the doctors, the 6/- was increased to 9/-. Of this, 6d. was taken from the Sanatorium Benefit Funds (abolished as a National Health Insurance benefit in 1921), and a new 2/6d. was found by the taxpayer. In this way contributions found seven-ninths of 6/6d.; and the Exchequer, 2/6d. plus two-ninths of 6/6d.; the resulting amounts show that the Exchequer two-ninths (the fraction paid for all other benefits) had already become four-ninths before the medical provisions of the Act had started. When additional amounts by way of temporary war bonus were paid to doctors and chemists, in the closing days of the War, these were found by the Exchequer.

Then came the demand for a definite increase in the remuneration of doctors and chemists, with arbitration in the case of the former. The total cost increased, as from the beginning of 1920, to 13/9d. Additional weekly insurance contributions, partly as a direct result of this increase, were imposed by the National Insurance Act of 1920, and by the same Act the cost of Medical Benefit was required to be met out of insurance funds to the extent of 9/6d., seven-ninths of this amount coming from contributions. The Exchequer continued to find the balance of the 13/9d. (4/3d.) as well as two-ninths of 9/6d.—a total of nearly 6/6d. out of 13/9d., or rather more than the four-ninths which the Exchequer had all along been paying, and more than double the share (two-ninths) which had been originally provided for in the Act of 1911.

A reduction in the remuneration of the doctors and the chemists was effected in 1922, the relief going entirely to the Exchequer; the Geddes Committee recommended that the Exchequer should be further relieved and should get back to the two-ninths basis laid down by the Act of 1911. The Government adopted this recommendation. The total cost of Medical Benefit—at any rate up to the end of 1923—having now become about 12/- a year, and 9/6d. only being provided for in the Act of 1920, the question arose whether Parliament should be asked to increase the weekly insurance contributions of the employer or the employed person, or both. The Consultative Council appointed by the Minister, which embodies approved society experience, advised that this should not be done at the time. They recommended that up to the end of 1923 the money required, over and above the statutory amount of 9/6d., should be found by drawing on the accumulated surpluses in the benefit funds of approved societies. The Government Actuary expressed the view that this could safely be done.

Effect was given to this proposal in the National Insurance Act, 1922, with a modification whereby an insurance fund under the control of the Department, called the Central Fund (primarily constituted for meeting deficiencies in approved societies' funds) reimbursed the benefit funds to the extent of one-third of the amount specially contributed by those funds. Thus, for the years 1922 and 1923 the sums available for the Medical Benefit were derived:—

> As to the main part (i.e., about 80 per cent. of the whole) from the contributions of employers and employed, to the extent of seven-ninths, and from the Exchequer to the extent of two-ninths:
>
> And as to the remainder (i.e., the other 20 per cent.), from the benefit funds of approved societies, as a temporary measure, those funds being reimbursed, however, to some extent from a central insurance fund and by the Exchequer.

For purposes of illustration, assuming the total cost of Medical Benefit in Great Britain to be nine million pounds, the cost was met approximately in the following proportions:—

	£
Employers..	3 millions
Employed	2¾ "
Exchequer..	2 "
Central and Benefit Funds	1¼ "
Total	9 millions

The provisions embodied in the 1922 Act, whereby temporary contributions in relief of State expenditure on Medical Benefit were made from the benefit funds of approved societies, gave rise to questionings on the subject of the future control of the service.

In the discussions during 1923 on the capitation fee, the societies sought to make it clear that they did not seek to control the medical service, but were jealous for the safety of the other benefits payable out of the National Health Insurance Fund. The doctors' representatives expressed the view that the cost of medical benefit should be met wholly out of that Fund, as a normal and necessary piece of Insurance expenditure, and that the Fund could quite well bear the charge for any liability reasonably likely to be incurred for the cost of Medical Benefit. In the result, provision was made in the Act of 1924 for meeting, for the three years 1924-6, the cost in excess of the 9/6d. provided for in the Act of 1920, out of the Central Fund and other special sources of income in the National Health Insurance Fund.

From 1927 onwards, the cost of Medical Benefit is directed to be met out of the National Health Insurance Fund, as previously urged by the doctors' representatives, and a sum of 13/- per annum is earmarked by statute for Medical Benefit, to include payments to doctors and chemists and expenses of administration. The contribution of the Exchequer towards the sum of 13/- is one-seventh in the case of men and one-fifth in the case of women.

Appendix No. 10.

Examination of the Report of the Medical Planning Commission

by R. W. Harris

(Reprinted from the British Medical Journal of 16th January, 1943.)

It was manifest from the outset that the labours of the Medical Planning Commission would not be restricted by its terms of reference, which were " to study wartime developments and their effect on the country's medical services both present and future." The Commission has proceeded to consider the whole question of the future of the medical services, whether as affected by wartime developments or otherwise. It is to be congratulated on an exceedingly interesting and well-balanced draft interim report, on the wisdom of publishing the report as a draft, and asking that it should be freely discussed by the profession. It is possible that the commentary of a layman—not without experience of administration—who has tried to keep himself informed of medical opinion over a period of years may be of some collateral value.

With the " broad definition of the objects of medical service in this country," as adopted by the Commission, there must be universal agreement. The differences of opinion begin when it is considered how the objects are to be attained.

The Case for Extension of N.H.I.

In paragraphs 47 and 48 of the draft report it is stated that the majority view is against a whole-time salaried Government service. It is contended that " the quality of individual service would not necessarily be improved by the replacement of a variable income by a fixed income or by the substitution of the State for the individual in the selection and employment of a doctor. . . . National Health Insurance has proved a greater success than was anticipated either by its supporters or by its opponents. . . . Its medical service contains features which have proved to be essentially sound, such as free choice of doctor, the minimum of interference by the State, and the central negotiation of terms and conditions of service."

As regards the question of the quality of the service being improved by the replacement of a variable income by a fixed income, it is surely unnecessary to say that no serious student of the subject has ever contended that an alteration in the method of remunerating the doctor would greatly affect the quality of the service which he gives. Has it not frequently been contended in support of the capitation system of payment under the N.H.I. scheme that a doctor will give as good a service when he is paid by a capitation fee as if paid a fee for each attendance or for each service rendered? But the question arises whether the objects of reform in medical practice as set out by the Commission are best attained and the best standard of medical service reached under a system of competition for patients, sale of practices, and all the financial troubles inherent in that system, particularly in the case of doctors wishing to establish themselves in practice. Criticisms offered by general practitioners themselves and summarized in the draft report form a grave indictment, but the gravity of the problem is by no means understated. The financial strain in many cases is becoming an increasingly serious menace to the efficiency of the medical practitioner.

Is it unfair to say that the medical profession has learned from industry the value of competition but has not to any large extent learned the value of organization? It is surely organization of medical practice which is necessary to procure the best results; the method of payment has not, or should not have, any real bearing on the question.

Employment of Doctor and Free Choice.

The phrase " the substitution of the State for the individual in the selection and employment of a doctor " has about it a disarming air of rhetoric. Under the National Health Insurance scheme there is no selection of doctors for employment in the service; every registered practitioner can enter the service by signing his name, and it requires the operation of a very formidable piece of machinery to secure his removal.

It cannot be seriously thought by critics of any scheme of organised national medical service that any responsible body of persons is going to propose that the "State," through the agency of, let us say, the Civil Service Commission, is to select the men to be engaged in the medical service. The proposal which would command the most general assent would be that set out in paragraph 52 of the report, whereby a Central Medical Services Board "predominantly medical in its composition" would have "executive functions in regard to the entry of the profession into the service." The statement about selection of the doctor by the individual—as opposed to selection by the State—is difficult to understand, but it presumably refers to the free choice of doctor, which is, in theory, one of the cardinal features of service under the National Health Insurance scheme.

Is there not in this matter a wide difference between theory and practice? No one would deny the value of the principle stated on medical grounds; equally no informed person would assert that it is a vital factor under the National Health Insurance scheme with more than a small proportion of the patients. There is a constant change of population. Large numbers of people probably move every few years, and when they come into a fresh district they are faced with the choice of a fresh doctor. Is it seriously contended that any large proportion of them choose their doctor on any other grounds than proximity or the casual advice of a neighbour? Then, again, is not the recognition of the capital value of practices, so that they are bought and sold, in direct conflict with the idea that insured persons display any anxiety about the particular doctor who should attend them? It is not open to question that, when a practice changes hands and the insured persons on the outgoing doctor's list are all notified they will automatically pass on to the list of the incoming doctor, unless they make a fresh choice, a quite insignificant number make such a fresh choice.

The right of a patient to choose his own doctor can be widely recognized under any scheme of national service, whether salaried or not, and there seems to be no inherent difficulty whatever in giving full play to the principle of free choice of doctor to the extent to which the choice is likely to be exercised. The experience of 30 years of insurance administration does not give any support to the view that a proportion of patients coming to a health centre would exercise the right of choice of doctor to such an extent as to create an embarrassment in the distribution of the patients among the doctors. At the outset, of course, there would have to be considered such questions as the right of the doctor coming under the scheme to bring with him, as it were, to the local centre his existing patients; indeed, this would be a common-sense beginning. If a doctor had an embarrassing number of patients, so that he would have an unfair share of the work, the difficulty could probably be met by informing the patients of the right they already enjoy to exercise a fresh choice. It may safely be predicted that the majority would have to be allocated, and naturally as many as possible would be left where they were.

Minimum of State Interference.

There is always the danger of a certain amount of prejudice being introduced into these discussions by the use of the word "State," with its implications of State interference with the proper and normal functions of doctors and of a cast-iron discipline and control undermining the doctor's efficiency. These can be avoided at the outset of the establishment of a national service by the proper organization of the central and local administration, so that the medical profession has a clear and definite voice in those matters which affect the personnel and the quality and kind of the services to be rendered; and especially in the organization of the services at the health centres and with the content of those services.

Is the profession really satisfied with the present complications involved in having to deal with the title to benefit of an insured person and with the disciplinary machinery, even though it admittedly does not function to any large extent, this again being due very largely to the apathy of the insured persons?

Scope of a National Service.

Those who press for the extension of the National Health Insurance medical service to the dependants of the present insured persons and to those of a "like economic status" often overlook the fact that the limit of £420 in the compulsory scheme is not a limit of total income, and that even as a limit of remuneration it does not apply to the great mass of the insured population—namely, those who are engaged in manual labour. The proposal bristles with such difficulties that it may well prove to be impracticable. Who is to decide? Are the income-tax authorities to come into the scheme? Can it be visualised what Parliament is likely to think of such a proposal?

And if an individual is held to be outside the scheme, is he to be debarred from the facilities afforded at the health centre, notwithstanding that as a tax-payer he has contributed to the cost? For in a national scheme, if gigantic complications and difficulties are to be avoided, there can be no datum line where people would cease to contribute towards the service. The health of the community is the first consideration of the community as a whole, and the time is not far distant when it will be recognised that everyone in the country must contribute to the service according to his ability to pay.

Would it be right or proper that one citizen should have some better kind of medical service than another, and is the citizen who is to be excluded from the benefits of the public service the one who, in fact, has made a larger contribution to the cost of the service than the citizen who is included? If the wealthy man has contributed to the medical service according to his ability to pay he must clearly be granted the right, whether he wishes to avail himself of it or not, to all the facilities that are provided by the service.

Custom and tradition count for a great deal, and in a period of transition there must remain a large amount of private practice gradually and slowly dying; but if the same doctor is to take part-time salaried service under the national scheme based on a publicly provided centre, and concurrently carry on private practice from his surgery, confused and chaotic problems will persist. It would be idle to gloss over the fact that, however long the transitional period may be—and it may well prove to be much longer in consultant and specialist practice than in the case of the general practitioner—the days of private practice would eventually come to an end. For private practice would mean the right of a doctor and patient to come to an understanding as to the fees to be paid for a service for which the patient has already paid in full and which cannot be better than the best.

During the transitional period questions of compensation will have to be settled, probably in each individual case, by a court of arbitration. Parliament may well regard as worth while a generous scheme of compensation as part of the price of getting the best

Central and Local Administration.

possible and most comprehensive service. This is not the place to examine the problems of compensation, but merely to recognize frankly that they are formidable. It is clear that a standing court of arbitration would have a long period of operations, dealing with individual cases in diminishing volume throughout the whole period of transition.

With regard to administration, there should be whole-hearted approval for two statements in paras. 51 and 52 of the report. One central authority should be concerned solely with all the civilian medical and auxiliary services of the country, and this authority must be responsible through a Minister to Parliament. The Minister in the exercise of his powers would require, for the wider problems of administration (especially those relating to the co-ordination of the work of the various local authorities), a secretariat with the necessary financial, registration, and accounting arrangements; but the "Central Medical Services Board which is predominantly medical in its composition" which is visualized (although as an alternative to another scheme) in para. 52 is one that would command general assent. This Board, it is proposed, in addition to advising the Minister, would have "executive functions in regard to the entry of the profession into the public medical service, disciplinary machinery, superannuation arrangements, and possibly postgraduate and refresher course arrangements."

With regard to local centres of administration, the local authorities of this country as at present constituted are already greatly overworked, and it is the trend of modern legislation continually to add to their burdens. The proposal to link the existing public health services, including hospital administration, with the new public medical service would mean that the existing local authorities would have to be closely associated with or represented on any new authority that was established. But it does not seem open to question that new local authorities with large areas should be set up, and that in the schemes for establishing these authorities something like the counterpart locally of the Central Medical Services Board should be reproduced.

The questions relating to central and local administration are of the highest importance, but when the controlling authority has been decided upon, what really matters is the quality of the service ultimately provided at the local centres—that is the work of the practitioner himself. The controlling authority may be very efficient and wisely constituted, but it is the "delivery of the goods" by the individual doctor that matters. Parliament will decide, but will be guided very largely by those who will have to "deliver the goods."

THE END.